Polymyalgia Rheumatica and Giant Cell Arteritis

A survival guide

3rd edition

Dr Kate Gilbert and Dr Vanessa Quick

with Dr Anne O'Brien

Published 2026 by Oberdan Books.

ISBN: 978-1-0666646-0-3

Oberdan Books, 54 Avondale Road, Wolverhampton, WV6 0AJ, UK

Dedication

To Keith and Tom

Praise for the second edition

"I am just so glad that this book was recommended to me by other sufferers of Polymyalgia Rheumatica on the HeathUnlocked forum. It has been like having a big sister who knows and CARES about the condition and is able to explain, comfort and advise. Kate writes clearly and honestly, from her position as an experienced long-term sufferer of the condition." Chrissie, UK.

"Recommended reading for those with PMR or GCA. The author covers a lot of things that doctors don't take the time to explain. Having GCA myself, I found it a very good resource and it answered a lot of my questions." Lynette, USA.

"This book is priceless in helping you understand what to expect and how to deal with having PMR. If I could give this book 10 stars, I would. Easy to read, great reference, and includes everything you need to know to manage your PMR." 'Itsnickers', USA.

"I've been looking forward to the publication of the third edition of this book very much. Previous editions have been so helpful to people suffering from PMR and GCA and all those who care about them or treat them." Dorothy Byrne, Patron, PMRGCAuk.

Foreword

I was delighted when Kate asked me to help her with the third edition of her book. However, there was a challenge ahead. How could I help with the content without moving the viewpoint away from the patient? It was very important that the book remained a book by Kate; in her clear, accessible, and engaging style, with topics of interest to Kate, as this was the great strength of the previous editions. I felt my role was not to replace her voice, but to support it, offering context where helpful, sharing current understanding, and my own perspective as a rheumatologist with specialist interest in PMR and GCA.

In some places, Kate has chosen to include short sections I have written to summarise my perspective, because she felt readers would value hearing this directly. However, in most instances, it felt more natural and helpful to weave these contributions into the updated main text, so that the narrative remains seamless and centred on her viewpoint.

In clinical research, the order of authorship carries meaning. The first author leads the work and contributes most directly to its creation. The last author provides guidance and support. In that spirit, I see Kate as the clear first author of this book. She has led it, shaped it, and given it its voice. I have been privileged to contribute alongside her in a supporting role.

I am very grateful to Kate for inviting me to share in this project, because I have gained not only a deeper appreciation of the patient experience, but also the pleasure of forming a valued friendship. I hope you enjoy reading it as much I have enjoyed helping to create it.

Dr Vanessa Quick

Contents

Prologue - Kate's story

This is how it happened for me. One morning, at the age of 54, I woke with a searing pain in my shoulders and a strange feeling of paralysis. I stared at the ceiling for a while feeling terrified, and then set about hauling myself out of bed. I crashed into the bedroom wall and sat down to think. "You've got polymyalgia rheumatica, like Mum had", I said to myself, as my memory dug up images of my mother dragging herself around 20 years before.

Having a long-term illness was not in my script. I thought I was doing all the right things; keeping fit, active, keeping the weight under control. However, one thing I had not been keeping under control as I got into my 50s was my level of stress. Looking back, I can see stress had been piling up on me from all directions. On the face of it, I had a wonderful life. As we know, stress isn't only caused by the bad things in life. Change that seems positive can also carry its burden of stress on the body and mind.

We had moved to Italy for my husband's job. It was all a wonderful adventure, and we as excited as a pair of newly-weds setting up our first home. We bought a new apartment near Milan and set about making it our "forever" home. It was just a concrete shell when we bought it, and all the work of creating the finishing, installing the plumbing, talking to builders, choosing floors and so on, fell to me, who had not a word of Italian before we started.

I would not change a minute of that experience, but I was not paying attention to the toll it was taking on my health. The month we moved in, my husband's company announced they wanted to change direction and his position was no longer secure. I needed to pick up my career again. I went back to the UK to work, as a head of department in a Midlands university. I wasn't a popular choice for the job. The department had a favoured internal candidate, and they weren't at all happy about getting me instead.

Two years of struggle and isolation followed, during which I was making the most of Ryanair's cheap fares by going home to Milan every couple of weeks to see my man, who was trying to set himself up with a new career. Somewhere in the middle of it all, our daughter gave birth to our first grandchild by Caesarean section after four gruelling days of labour.

We took an Easter holiday in Umbria to recharge our batteries. It was so cold and wet that I contracted a bout of viral pneumonia. Everything seemed to be going wrong. We lived from day to day, coping. Looking back, it is not surprising I got ill and my immune system went into overdrive.

Immediately following diagnosis of polymyalgia rheumatica, the prednisolone had me jumping around like a budgie on Trill. Just two hours after my first dose I ran up the stairs. I felt reborn, and full of energy. Four weeks in, and a colleague found me in my office, weeping uncontrollably. I seemed to have hit a brick wall. On his insistence, I called the surgery and said, "I need to see a doctor. I can't stop crying and I don't know why." To their great credit, the surgery told me to go round straight away. When the doctor asked me the classic depression question, "Have you had any thoughts of harming yourself?" I realised how low I had been, without being fully aware of it. She signed me off for a month. I crawled into bed with my grandson's teddy and stayed there for a week. My husband came over from his job in Italy to look after me and never went back. I was off work for one month, but frankly, it should have been three. I had an interview with Occupational Health. No, they had not heard of polymyalgia rheumatica. But they could get me a counsellor. The single most effective thing the counsellor said to me was to stop trying to change others, and start looking after myself.

I had felt from a very young age that somehow it was my responsibility to make things right, to make things better. But from that moment, I changed my attitude towards work. The most important thing was to help myself back to health, and to still be there for my family.

I wasn't a typical PMR patient in the rheumatology textbook sense. I continued to be in pain while on steroids, and to suffer from stiffness. I did however manage to carry on working and look after my baby grandson for three days a week, neither of which would have been possible without the medication. I spent a couple of years stuck on a moderate daily dose of steroids without being able to reduce. Two years in, and feeling desperate, I looked for support. And that was the start of the adventure that would become PMRGCAuk.

Ten years after my diagnosis, and fully recovered from PMR, I started to write about everything I had learned from working and sharing with rheumatologists, researchers, and, above all, fellow patients. This book is the latest part of the story.

1 Introduction

Have you just received a diagnosis of polymyalgia rheumatica or giant cell arteritis? If so, I'm willing to bet you're feeling confused and apprehensive. Wouldn't it be just your luck to find yourself with a disease nobody in your family or circle of friends has heard of, with the prospect of taking steroid pills for a long time? And all that on top of feeling, frankly, pretty rough. Allow me to sit you down with this book and give you all the information you need and whatever reassurance I can offer. Let this book be a companion on your journey towards recovery.

Here in one place, you will find explanations of what PMR and GCA are, how they are diagnosed and treated, and how you can best approach being on steroid medications for a considerable length of time. We will give you insights into current research, developments in imaging techniques which are opening new frontiers of understanding, and a perspective on new medications that could present (at least partial) alternatives to steroids. We will focus on answers to those inevitable questions you will have on what you can do to help yourself towards recovery.

This edition follows ten years on from the last, which became a world bestseller. I chose a self-publishing platform because for me it was essential that anyone, anywhere in the world should be able to get hold of a copy within days, and this precious information shouldn't end up on a remaindered table and then pulped, as happens to so many books.

Given the book is obviously so valuable to patients (just check out the online reviews) and because it is now twenty years since I fell ill with PMR, the need for a third edition presented a challenge. How to make sure it is really up-to-date and the friendly tone of the writing also delivers some cast-iron information and advice? Challenge also presented opportunity. Why not invite collaboration with a clinical rheumatologist? I was delighted when

Dr Vanessa Quick, who is also a trustee of PMRGCAuk, came forward full of enthusiasm for the project and agreed to co-author sections. Vanessa sees lots of patients with PMR and GCA, she contributes to practice-based research, and she's passionate about medical education.

I tried very hard to keep everything in the second edition evidence based. Now, with Vanessa's collaboration, we have been stricter about this. So, you won't find any endorsements of diets where there is no research evidence of effectiveness. You won't find recommendations for herbal remedies or advice on how to manage your pain with alternative therapies. This is not because we rule them out of hand, but simply, the proper scientific evidence for their effectiveness is not available, as the necessary studies have not been carried out and published in the scientific literature.

This introductory chapter gives a brief overview of polymyalgia rheumatica (PMR) and giant cell arteritis (GCA); explaining briefly what they are and why they go together in the same book. I then take you through the rest of the content and point out what has been updated and changed from the last edition.

Even though they are among the most common rheumatological diseases impacting older people, polymyalgia rheumatica and giant cell arteritis are not well known by the public. It may have taken you months, and many rounds of tests, to finally get a diagnosis. You don't know how you are going to be, or how your health condition is going to affect your life. You will need reliable information and advice to manage your condition and keep on top of your symptoms while avoiding, as much as you can, the unwanted effects of steroid treatment.

You may be feeling lousy right now because you are in the early stages and are only now getting used to the idea of having a long-term inflammatory illness. The first thing you need to know about PMR and GCA is that you have an excellent chance of getting better. Many people are able to complete their course of steroid medication within two years or so and move on without too much difficulty. With luck, this will be you. It used to be received wisdom that PMR and GCA are self-limiting diseases, burning themselves out in a couple of years[1]. Research of recent years has shown this isn't the case for a sizable proportion of patients, who may be on medication for considerably longer. Maybe you have reached for this book because you're one of them and you want to find a way through. Whatever your situation turns out to be, we hope this book will answer your questions going forward.

I used to feel guilty meeting other people with PMR and GCA through my work with PMRGCAuk, telling them I was now recovered. I imagined they might feel resentful, thinking "oh, it's alright for her". But instead, it seems most people are only too glad to meet someone who is a PMR or GCA survivor.

I call this book a survival guide, not because your life is in danger, but because you are going to be dealing with a long-term condition incompletely understood even by specialists, and it's not clear what the outcome will be. You are probably going to feel sometimes as though you are fighting a dragon; a fiery, fierce, unpredictable creature that can rear its head again when you think you have beaten it. You may well encounter health professionals who seem to know very little about your condition. Your friends and family might act completely bewildered to hear you have something they have never heard of. Many days can feel like a battle. Our very first group of patients who got together to set up a national support organisation in the UK called ourselves the "PMRFighters" because we felt we were combating ignorance and complacency, as well as a nasty rheumatological condition.

You and your dragon

The idea of a duel with a dragon came to me one day when I was thinking about the challenge of managing a long-term condition, and at the same time managing the tapering of the steroid medication. Imagine being tied up against a rock, your limbs unable to move because of the ropes. You're facing a dragon with terrifying, staring eyes, breathing fire and smoke, consuming everything standing in its way. This dragon is out to get you.

The fiery head is like the acute phase when we first fall ill with PMR or GCA. We're consumed by inflammation. We feel helpless and horribly ill. Then, see how the dragon has a long, sloping, spiny back, going up and down with spikes? It is like the long period when we are trying to recover, "tapering" the steroids, and perhaps having difficulty, with one flare-up after another. We hope your personal dragon will soon be tamed, but we can't promise. The dosage of medication goes up and down, our symptoms go up and down, and finding the right balance between the two can be a struggle. Now see the dragon's tail. This has a sharp point that could take you by surprise. Just when you thought you had your old dragon beaten, up comes the tail to strike you. Wallop! Here is the sting in the tail of PMR or GCA. The years on steroids, and the burden of the illness itself, might leave you with an unwelcome reminder, in the form of injuries to your tendons and ligaments, thinning of the bones, adrenal insufficiency, or perhaps Type 2 diabetes.

The trick with the dragon is to manage the risks at each stage of the battle, whether you're dealing with the head, the long spiky back, or the tail. We hope your GP or rheumatologist can take the role of the knight in shining armour who helps out. But *you* are going to be the hero or heroine of your story and sort out your dragon one way or another. You are going to need information to keep one step ahead. That's why you need this survival guide.

Separate but connected

If you have either PMR or GCA, you might wonder why both are covered in this book. Polymyalgia rheumatica (PMR) and giant cell arteritis (GCA, occasionally known as temporal arteritis, or TA) have traditionally been regarded as separate illnesses. Although they have long been known to be associated, the factors that determine how and why patients develop one or the other are still not fully understood. PMR presents with pain around the joints attaching our limbs to our bodies. This pain tends to be felt in the muscles and structures around the joints, rather than the joints themselves. Imaging shows inflammation in the structures around the joints such as the *bursas*, or fluid sacs, which cushion the joints, and the tendons anchoring our muscles to our skeleton. There may be general malaise, perhaps fever, and fatigue. GCA may present too with these symptoms, and often acute head sensations in the form of headaches, tender scalp, or jaw pain. But the site of the inflammation in GCA is the walls of the arteries taking blood around the body.

Both conditions affect older people, rarely affecting people under 50 years old, raising the question of how they may be related to the ageing process itself. The overlaps have long been evident, leading experts to suggest they are different manifestations of the same spectrum disorder. In the UK, there are about 40,000 new cases of PMR and 10,000 new cases of GCA a year.

About one in ten people with PMR is also diagnosed with GCA, while approximately half of people with GCA also have the symptoms of PMR. They can happen together, overlap, or appear one after the other, so it's helpful to understand both.

What *is* polymyalgia rheumatica?

PMR is a common disorder, affecting about 1 in 50 people over their lifetime (2% of us)[2]. Translated into ordinary language, the term *polymyalgia rheumatica* means "muscle pain all over the place". This describes some of the symptoms, though not very accurately. But it doesn't explain what the illness actually *is*.

Although you may never have heard of PMR before, in medical terms it is common. The British Society for Rheumatology and the British Health Professionals in Rheumatology published guidelines for the management of PMR in the UK, in 2010[2]. These open with: "PMR is the most common inflammatory rheumatic disease in the elderly and is one of the biggest indications for long-term steroid therapy. There are difficulties in diagnosis, with heterogeneity in presentation, response to steroids and disease course." This is actually the closest these guidelines get to a definition. Although a large-scale international project published recommendations in 2015[3], we are well overdue some updated guidelines for the medical profession in the UK. It's good to know these are currently underway for both PMR and GCA.

Carole, aged 71 at the time she was diagnosed with PMR, gives a vivid and classic description of the sudden onset of paralysing stiffness that heralds PMR:

> *"I woke one morning feeling almost paralysed with stiffness and pain, particularly in my arms and hands.*
>
> *"After around half an hour of trying to get out of bed, by placing my bent knees over the side of the bed and gently lowering them to the bedroom floor, I then had the problem of getting to my feet, standing, and walking.... I felt there was no strength in my arms to push myself up to stand, and no strength in my leg muscles to get me up from my knees. I crawled from beside the bed to the central heating radiator to pull myself up to stand.*
>
> *"In total, it took me an hour from being laid in bed to my feet! What had caused this and what was it? I had felt perfectly OK before that morning."*

This sudden onset is typical, although it's also common for patients to look back and realise they had been feeling under par for some time beforehand.

The use of the term "elderly" to describe people who get PMR is interesting, and controversial. It is true the average age of onset is about 72. But averages can be misleading. PMR actually generally strikes people over the age of 50, being very rare, as we have said, but not entirely unknown, among people under 50. People in their fifties or sixties do not consider themselves elderly, and the word tends to evoke a stereotype in the minds of many clinicians about what the typical patient is like. “Elderly” conjures up images of storybook grandmas with glasses and grey hair in buns, of crocheted shawls and sensible shoes. It negates the experience of thousands of people in their 50s and 60s who develop PMR and GCA while they are still working, vigorous and feeling in their prime. It feeds into a general perception these conditions don’t matter so much as others, like rheumatoid arthritis, because they affect people who are in decline in any case. I also suspect it has an effect on how interesting PMR has been seen to be among doctors.

Medical consensus is that PMR is an autoimmune inflammatory illness. The immune system has become overactive and out of control, creating excessive inflammation in various parts of the body.

Your doctor may have told you PMR is a condition of the muscles. And the term “myalgia” does mean muscle pain. Certainly, if you have PMR you feel intense pain in your muscles, perhaps in your shoulders or the tops of your arms. However, scans seem to show the inflammation appearing to concentrate in the *musculoskeletal structures* around the major joints.

What *is* giant cell arteritis?

Giant cell arteritis is a *vasculitis,* an inflammatory disease of the circulation system[4]. We have all heard of arthritis, but few people outside medicine have ever heard of *art-er-it-is*. The “-itis” bit means inflammation. In the case of GCA, we are talking about inflammation of the arteries, not *arthritis,* which means inflammation of the joints. If you are going to be ill with something for two years or more, you might as well know how to pronounce it properly. To be honest, doctors are not very good at checking whether their patients have actually understood the name of their illness.

It is even more confusing because, surprisingly, GCA falls into the category of rheumatoid or musculoskeletal illness, rather than the category of vascular illness, or illness of the blood circulation system. Don't rheumatologists deal with rheumatoid arthritis? Yes! So just remember this is art-*er*-it-is, and tell all your family and friends how to pronounce it, explain it means inflammation of the arteries, and instruct them on no account ever to ask you, "How's your arthritis?". It might be helpful to rethink your idea of what a rheumatologist does - basically, they are a specialist in inflammation[5].

What happens in GCA is that the walls of the large arteries become stuffed full of extra inflammatory cells, making the artery wall thick and puffy. Artery walls are in fact complex organs, consisting of three layers. Imagine cutting an artery across so you can see a cross section. Normally the wall is thin like a wedding ring, but in GCA it can be so thick it looks more like a ring doughnut. Some of these inflammatory cells may be strange giant cells, which, compared with normal cells, really are giants. It is like comparing a child's birthday balloon with an airbed. The process by which these massive cells form is complicated, but they are very specific to GCA and give the condition its name.

The danger is that these inflamed walls can narrow the inner channel of the artery and cut off the blood supply to key parts of the body, particularly the eyes or the brain. Generally, because there is a good network of blood vessels into the head, the blood manages to find a way through that is not blocked, and so all the parts of the head – brain, ears, mouth, nose and the eyes, can get an adequate supply. This is why people will often notice other symptoms before noticing any serious interference with their vision.

The most common symptom of giant cell arteritis is a new type of persistent pain somewhere in the head, a signal of inflammation. This pain may be acute and throbbing and tender to touch. There are many more common causes of pain in the head, as we all know. Infection, such as a cold or flu, bright sunlight, stress, a cricked neck or too much wine the night before, can all trigger a nasty headache. Other conditions can present very much like GCA, and this might be a clue as to why younger people (in their 40s) are sometimes initially suspected of having GCA. But GCA is, without doubt, predominantly a disease of older people where the vast majority are actually over 60.

GCA is, in fact, the most common vasculitis among people over 50, and it is most prominent among people of North European descent. It has been estimated that by the year 2050, there will be around 3 million people in North America, Europe, and Oceania (Australasia and the South Pacific) diagnosed with GCA. Of these, it's estimated half a million will experience sight impairment[6].

GCA and vision loss

Things really start to look bad (literally) when visual disturbance comes into the picture. If the blood supply to the optic nerve is severely reduced, the most serious and common cause of vision loss is Anterior Ischaemic Optic Neuropathy (AION). Another, less common but equally serious cause is Central Retinal Artery Occlusion (CRAO), where the main artery supplying the retina becomes blocked. Each is effectively a stroke in the eye. The vision damage caused can be total and is usually irreversible. This blindness usually occurs suddenly, over minutes to hours, but some people have warning symptoms or stepwise worsening over a few days before the permanent vision loss becomes established. You might experience blurring, or double vision. Occasionally the vision in one eye might fail altogether for a little while and then come back intermittently. This is the cardinal danger sign for GCA and is a signal to you to get immediate medical help, by going to

A&E if necessary (ER in the US). In every case, it is a medical emergency and if the doctor is concerned about the probability of sight loss from GCA, then treatment should be started as soon as possible.

Unfortunately, about one in five people with GCA experience sight loss before diagnosis, or during the process of diagnosis. Many of these are people who put off going to the doctor because they don't want to waste the doctor's time. This is why it's important for older people and those around them to know the key signs and symptoms of GCA. Once you are on treatment, taking steroids, the risk of sight loss reduces dramatically with each day of treatment, and is very rare once someone has been on steroids for a few weeks. If you are newly diagnosed, you can have some reassurance, but it's still best to stay vigilant.

The missing link?

Many people with GCA also have PMR and might have had undiagnosed PMR for some time before their GCA diagnosis. Conversely, having PMR increases the risk of getting GCA. There are different schools of thought about what the connection is precisely. Advances in imaging techniques have shed some light, but things still aren't cut and dried.

In GCA, it is the larger arteries around the head and neck, and sometimes the major blood vessels supplying the arms that are most affected. Recent research has shown the primary site of inflammation in PMR appears to be in a range of tissue types, including tendons and fluid sacs, around the joints. So not primarily inside the joints (which might point to rheumatoid arthritis) and not in the arteries (which would point towards vasculitis). However, the typical inflammation of structures around joints that we see in PMR can also be seen in many GCA patients, and even those who don't also have PMR symptoms, which suggests they might have "sub-clinical" PMR rumbling away in the background. And similarly, some people with PMR may have sub-clinical inflammation of their large arteries. Sub-clinical means a disease is present, but not causing symptoms that the patient is feeling. It's evident there is significant overlap and blurring about what is happening in each illness.

Increasingly, some specialists believe that evidence from imaging techniques points to this being a spectrum condition, with different manifestations but a shared underlying disorder[7]. Both diseases affect older people, both have general symptoms of illness as well as their specific unique symptoms, both show imbalances of the same inflammatory chemicals in the bloodstream, especially one called IL-6, and both show a remarkable response to steroid treatment[8].

This has led to the suggestion of a new name - GPSD, or *giant cell arteritis/PMR spectrum disease),* a term gradually gaining currency in rheumatology around the world (although you probably won't find your doctor using it yet). How it will be defined is currently going through a process of discussion and verification amongst experts, and we don't know yet whether the concept will be generally accepted in the scientific community. It has limitations, plenty of specialists have reservations about it, and we'll talk more about those later, but I find it intriguing, because it helps to illuminate the mystery of the connection between these two conditions, with the concept of an underlying disorder, showing different manifestations and different approaches to treatment.

About this book

That reinforcement of many people's hunch about the connection between PMR and GCA is one major reason I decided to bring out a third edition. Many messages from the second edition remain, but I've reorganised things to consider PMR and GCA in the same chapters on diagnosis and treatment, rather than addressing them separately.

The first edition came out in 2014. I was ten years on from the diagnosis of PMR and heavily involved with establishing and growing the charity PMRGCAuk. The second, expanded, edition followed in 2016 and has sold thousands of copies around the world. There is clearly a need for accessible information among the people who find themselves having to deal with PMR and GCA, and an appetite for something deeper than an introductory leaflet. In the subsequent years, besides the spectrum idea, a few important changes have taken place. These include advances in drug treatment of GCA, advances in imaging technology to understand each condition, and better understanding of the need for more personalised approaches to treatment with steroids and other steroid-sparing immune treatments for both GCA and PMR.

We have also lived through the traumatic period of Covid and the impact it had on health services around the world. It has probably changed how you communicate with your GP – much more likely to be a telephone call these days. We focus particularly on the UK's National Health Service, as this book is written primarily for a British readership. At the time of writing there is general consensus that the service is under immense strain, and we are still reeling from the impact of Covid on our services. We try to temper our calls for improved services such as ultrasound for everyone and rapid introduction of improved drugs with clear-eyed realism about the actual situation facing patients and doctors.

Support systems are so much better now, particularly in the UK. Ten years ago, PMRGCAuk was a new kid on the charity block, working hard to gain recognition, especially within the clinical world, and learning step by step how to provide support to patients and their families and carers. It has gone from strength to strength, and I'm pleased to give you more information about how it can support you. Patients have changed too. Twelve years ago, we were constantly hearing the litany that older people didn't use the internet. Well, the situation has completely changed now.

Sales of the second edition in the United States and Canada were initially surprising, and it was wonderful to receive messages of thanks and appreciation for the book from people on the other side of the pond. Vanessa and I are not qualified to tailor the content to your needs if you are not in the UK, but on the other hand we have tried to recognise our readership abroad in the choice of vignettes and patient stories we have included. International guidelines apply across North America and Europe. It's also helpful and interesting to know how the diseases are treated in other parts of the world, in other healthcare funding systems.

Many patients have a strong conviction that alternative therapies will help them recover. Vanessa and I are incidentally both of the view that, regrettably, alternative therapies do not have a great deal to offer in the treatment of PMR and GCA. Despite searching, we have not been able to find independent, unbiased evidence for alternative therapies working here. You may hate the drugs, but in this case, you need them, especially in the early stages. The people with PMR who manage to get through without steroid medication are few and far between. This is not to deny, though, that some therapies, such as massage, might help your wellbeing as you recover, and so we give some attention to them in the chapter on helping yourself to recovery. But any benefit you get from alternative therapies will be personal to you, and not generalisable to the whole population of people with PMR and GCA.

We are grateful to all the patients on PMRGCAuk's online forum HealthUnlocked[9] for PMR and GCA who are so generous in sharing their own stories. Here you will find lots of examples of experimentation with therapies and medication routines. Recent years have seen a surge of participation in the forum, and this has helped to create a huge bank of patient experience to inform understanding of what it's actually like having these conditions.

The second edition carried several sections and pages on the risk of sight loss posed by undiagnosed GCA. So much so that one or two online reviews suggested it was alarmist. This was never the intention. But ten years ago, PMRGCAuk was in the thick of a major campaign to inform the public and persuade health providers to put fast-track diagnosis systems into place. I had visited the Royal National Institute for the Blind in 2011 and had to explain to them what GCA was.

Today's situation is different. While not standard practice all over the country, there are many fast-track pathways for GCA operating and they are having a positive effect on the number of sight loss occurrences in GCA. This isn't to say the problem has gone away. I wrote in 2016 of my dream of eradicating GCA-related sight loss within ten years. We're not there yet, but we are moving in the right direction.

Another GCA-related change, linked to diagnosis, is the way ultrasound imaging techniques have taken over from the temporal artery biopsy as the gold standard method for diagnosis in the UK and Europe. Although there are still many places where quick access to ultrasound isn't available, it's greatly to be welcomed that the surgical procedure of biopsy is now a lot less necessary. Biopsies are still the first line test in the United States, perhaps because of the way the healthcare system is structured there, but this is changing too.

For years I have thought that to regard PMR and GCA just as rheumatic conditions is missing an important point. We have to look closer, and deeper, at what is happening inside our bodies. These are *autoimmune* conditions. The inflammation causing our pain is not due to wear and tear, nor to trauma or injury, but to the normally healthy processes of the immune system. When the immune system gets out of control, can't turn itself off and goes into overdrive, we suffer conditions linked to chronic inflammation. Autoimmune illnesses can affect any part of the body, from the muscles and joints, or the skin and connective tissue, to the gastric system. Perhaps it is a lottery which of these illnesses we fall prey to. We might count ourselves lucky we "only" get GCA or PMR. There is no smoke without fire, so having one autoimmune illness is probably an indicator there might be others lurking around the corner. Thus, how you manage your gradual recovery can pay dividends for your future health. Recovering well is a central theme of this book.

Structure and contents

Chapter 2 focuses on the diagnosis and early treatment of polymyalgia rheumatica and giant cell arteritis. There are key differences in the approach medicine takes, because GCA is a medical emergency, and PMR isn't.

We explain the processes and challenges of diagnosing PMR and GCA, and why steroid drugs, particularly prednisolone (prednisone in the US) are the first lines of treatment. We describe what to expect if you are sent for ultrasound scanning and/or a temporal artery biopsy.

We move on in Chapter 3 to the thorny issue of medication, particularly the issue of being on steroids for quite long periods of time. You will come across the terms *glucocorticoids*, *corticosteroids* and *steroids*, both in this book and your dealings with doctors. But essentially, here, they all mean the same thing. The chapter deals with how steroids work, and their possible effects on the body.

This can be a hard time for many sufferers, not least because the standard steroid treatment has the effect of filling out all our wrinkles and giving a lovely bloom to our skin. "NHS Botox" I've heard it called. It is confusing and, frankly, wearing, to have friends and family exclaim "Oh you do look well!" when you are feeling like crawling under a stone and not coming out again.

Chapter 4 is about the challenges of tapering your steroid dose, while staying on top of the worst symptoms of the conditions. We look at differences in tapering between GCA and PMR and face up to these conditions being "flaring" diseases. If you have PMR and are experiencing difficulties, we consider whether and how you might expect a referral to rheumatology.

Nowadays, PMR and GCA are described in the literature as "relapsing" diseases. Many of us experience a sudden or creeping return of symptoms, signs, and inflammation while on pred.

While clinicians usually refer to this as relapse, patients call it a flare. A relapse to a doctor means a return of symptoms *while you're still on treatment*, as well as after you stop. This is all quite confusing. From now on, when we talk about a return of symptoms while on steroids, we're going to go with the patients, and call it a flare, except where we need to use doctor-speak. "Flare" is more colourful, more in line with our fight-with-the-dragon metaphor and accurately describes how it feels to you and me.

In Chapter 5, we consider medications that might help reduce the dose of steroid needed. We focus on those steroid-sparing drugs in use for some time, and the potential of new "biologic" drugs. These offer a revolution in the treatment of chronic inflammatory conditions, especially where flares are common.

Chapter 6 tackles the impact on our lives of having these conditions and helping ourselves towards recovery. How do we find our own path to being the most well we can be? You need, while you are reading this book and through the course of your journey with GCA and PMR, to keep repeating the mantra "I am getting better". We need to learn to take the long view and believe in the body's power to heal itself. Because that is what it is doing. We can make it easier or harder for ourselves, and this is about making it easier.

Chapter 7 takes a separate look at exercise and activity. We are delighted that, for this section, we've been joined by Dr Anne O'Brien, who wrote her PhD thesis on physiotherapy and PMR.

Anne is Reader in Physiotherapy in the School of Allied Health Professions and Pharmacy, at Keele University, Staffordshire, UK.

Chapter 8 focuses on the forms of support you can access to help, and you might find you're even inspired to help others. The best way you could show your appreciation of this book is to become a member of PMRGCAuk!

Information is backed up with published sources listed in the References section. To begin with, I avoided academic conventions with numerous references. However, feedback indicated some readers would appreciate knowing more about the sources, and in this edition there are more. Some of our sources are freely available online, although not all medical journals are accessible to the public. So, if you see a small number next to the text, it points to a source listed in the reference section at the back of the book, where you can find more information if you wish. We have also included a glossary of terms for quick reference. Another addition has been the inclusion of several more stories from readers about their journey with PMR and GCA.

Where we wanted to include Vanessa's professional knowledge and experience in her own words, as if you were in the room with her, we have included a section headed "Vanessa says". This is presented in a different italicised font from the main text, to make it clear. There are 16 of these sections. However, I want to stress that her contribution as a consultant rheumatologist, specialising in vasculitis, runs throughout the main text as well. We have learned a lot from working together. Through long sessions of discussion and painstaking joint editing, we have crafted something unique – a book combining up-to-date medical knowledge while still keeping the experience of you, the patient, at the centre.

Enjoy the read!

2 Diagnosis & starting treatment

Polymyalgia rheumatica and giant cell arteritis have only relatively recently been recognised and defined by medicine. Before doctors realised these conditions were distinct from other painful and debilitating diseases, and before the advent of steroid therapy, there must have been a great deal of suffering. In van Eyck's 15th century painting "The Virgin and Child with Canon van der Paele"[10], we can see the poor canon had severely swollen and prominent arteries visible on his temple, and the severity of his headaches can only be imagined. As for polymyalgia rheumatica, it is only in very recent times that medicine has taken the aches and pains of old age seriously, realising ageing bones and muscles don't necessarily have to be agonisingly uncomfortable, and debilitation and general unwellness don't have to be an inevitable feature of later life. PMR was first recorded as "senile rheumatic gout" in 1888 and given the name polymyalgia rheumatica in the 1950s to recognise that the way it causes pain is diffused into diverse parts of the body[11].

We begin with PMR, simply because it affects more people than GCA, yet has been more of a medical mystery. If you have GCA, we recommend you still read through the whole chapter rather than jumping to the GCA diagnosis section, because much of the background information will apply to you too. Many people with GCA also have background PMR-type symptoms either before, at the same time, or after GCA has affected them.

Identifying and classifying PMR

PMR was first *systematically* observed and defined by a case report of 11 patients at Mount Sinai Hospital in New York, in 1966. Since then, various approaches have developed, and there used to be considerable discrepancy in how it was defined and identified in different countries. The PMR classification study, carried out by the American College of Rheumatology (ACR) and the European

League Against Rheumatism (EULAR), surveyed 111 rheumatologists and 53 non-rheumatologists in North America and Western Europe[12]. This survey was designed to boil down the various criteria clinicians use around the world to a manageable set everybody could agree on. This meant carefully weeding out those criteria that are not sufficiently well-represented across all cases of PMR. This was tremendously important, because it opened the doors to international research and the possibility of comparing research results across different studies, knowing that when they are talking about PMR, everybody is talking about the same thing. The study started with no less than 68 potential criteria and progressively narrowed them down to seven.

The Magnificent Seven are:

a. The person is aged 50 or over
b. Symptoms have lasted at least two weeks
c. Aching of both shoulders and/or pelvic girdle aching (the bilateral aspect is very important)
d. Morning stiffness lasting at least 45 minutes
e. An elevated erythrocyte sedimentation rate (ESR)
f. An elevated C-reactive protein level in the blood (CRP)
g. Rapid response to steroids.

All the clinicians and scientists agreed these should be included as the key classification criteria. It is worth noting one or two of the criteria that did not quite make the cut. There was a high level of agreement (84%) for including limitation of shoulder movement, and slightly lower agreement (76%) for including restricted hip mobility. Peripheral symptoms such as carpal tunnel syndrome and tenosynovitis were eliminated from the criteria. These also appear in some cases of PMR but not in sufficient numbers to warrant including them in the criteria for defining the disease. It's also worth noting here that the ESR and CRP tests aren't specific for PMR. In other words, these scores can indicate many other inflammatory illnesses. It remains the case, frustratingly, that there isn't a single blood or other test to definitively identify PMR.

Each of the Magnificent Seven classification criteria for PMR merits a closer look.

Aged 50 or over

Does this mean if you are younger than 50 you cannot have PMR? Well, not exactly, although it does give an indication of how rare it is in younger people. The average age of onset of PMR is 72. This leads doctors to believe it has a connection with the ageing process, or *senescence*. However, the fact is that in any distribution curve, there will be people at the extreme ends, the outliers who aren't typical. The range is huge, from people who are in the prime of life, strong, fit and active, to people who are already frail in later life.

I found it very difficult, in my mid-50s, to come to terms with having an illness old people are supposed to get. I hadn't even really got used to thinking of myself as middle-aged. I had been feeling full of beans and pretty fit.

For the unlucky few who do get PMR in their early 50s, doctors are unwilling to diagnose PMR unless they are quite certain all other possibilities have been eliminated. It is more likely an alternative diagnosis would be correct. The reluctance to diagnose is because putting people onto a course of steroids for two years or longer is an extremely serious matter, even when steroids are the right treatment. In the case of a young person wrongly diagnosed with PMR, the steroids will probably mask the symptoms of something else, potentially more sinister, going on.

As chair of PMRGCAuk, I heard several reports online and in patient support groups of people in their forties being diagnosed by their GPs. Discussion among some online patient groups gave the impression there were quite a lot of people being diagnosed younger than 50, whereas rheumatologists were assuring me this was very rare. I was sufficiently concerned to set up a straw poll among members of the internet forum, asking people how old they were when they got their diagnosis. Of 269 people who responded, 11, or 4%, were in the age group 45-49, and none were younger than 45. We knew it was the younger people who were more likely to be posting online, so we could assume that in the whole population diagnosed with PMR, perhaps 3% at the most would be younger than 50.

I also invited people who had diagnoses in their forties to share their story. Tracy, from the south-east of England and diagnosed at 46, is a typical example. Tracy says she was probably having symptoms for a couple of years before her diagnosis. She says successive visits to her GP didn't help until she saw a new doctor:

> *"In January I luckily made an appointment with a female doctor. I walked in, in a flood of tears, and she was amazing. She initially thought fibromyalgia but wanted to run some tests first. When I went back my ESR etc. were high and she did say although I am at the younger end of the scale, she was convinced then with the weakness it was polymyalgia, she put me on steroids and told me to go back five days later. When I went back feeling so much better, that confirmed it to her."*

This story of using the response to steroids to clinch the diagnosis makes me quite uncomfortable. Like Tracy, every single person under 50 who responded to me had been diagnosed by a GP, and not a rheumatologist. And not a single one had been referred to rheumatology either.

What do rheumatologists think about this? I asked some of the top researching experts on PMR in the world. Professor Eric Matteson, of the Mayo Clinic in the US, said he has had people younger than 50 referred to him, but in every case apart from one, he was able to find an alternative diagnosis that fitted the patient better. In other words, in all his decades-long career as a leading specialist on PMR in the USA, he had only ever seen one case of PMR in someone in their forties. On the other hand, he didn't maintain PMR is impossible or could never occur in a younger person.

Professor Bhaskar Dasgupta also says, "such persons should be diagnosed only after specialist review, never only in primary care." And Professor Marco Cimmino in Italy, although he says he has seen five such cases in his career, has only felt confident in diagnosis after performing a PET/CT scan on the patient. Dr Sarah Mackie reminds us that quite a few other diseases, not only rheumatological, can present with "polymyalgic" symptoms, so it is really important younger patients are seen by a specialist to rule this out. For example, certain forms of arthritis such as rheumatoid arthritis and psoriatic arthritis may have symptoms looking very much like GCA or PMR at first sight and are much more common in younger people than GCA or PMR.

You might still get the impression from discussions on the internet (e.g. Facebook groups) that members of patient groups are wedded to the idea of there being lots of people younger than 50 with PMR and GCA. In terms of absolute numbers there may be several, but as a proportion of the total population of patients, they are rare. I can only plead with group admins to be highly circumspect and join me and Vanessa in urging anyone under 55 who gets a diagnosis of PMR to take a copy of the latest BSR guidelines to a meeting with their doctor[13]. And whatever your age, don't allow a GP to conclude that your response to steroids is proof of the diagnosis. Almost anything will feel better if you take steroids for it, and the steroids will mess up your baseline blood results. By the time you have been on them for a few weeks, it will probably be too late for a rheumatologist to make an informed diagnosis until you are weaned off the steroids and have to start the whole process over again.

For this and other reasons, if you are younger than 55 and diagnosed with PMR by your GP, I would strongly recommend you push for a referral to hospital, for the very simple reason your age makes you an atypical patient, and it is quite likely the diagnosis may be mistaken. The added bonus of seeing a rheumatologist is that they are the specialist doctors who look after all these conditions, so you will be in the right hands regardless. There may well be resistance to this, as not all NHS rheumatologists agree that seeing younger PMR patients is necessary or that they have the capacity to see them. One possible way round this is to discuss with your doctor the possibility of referring you for investigation into EIA (early inflammatory arthritis) rather than PMR, especially if your local trust has an EIA diagnostic pathway that could get you seen quickly. If you can manage without steroids until you get an appointment, so much the better.

Symptoms lasting at least two weeks

Sometimes people have been suffering for ages before they go to the doctor and cannot even remember when it all started. Others have tried all kinds of remedies, or have suffered in silence, believing themselves to be afflicted with the aches and pains of growing older. PMR is much more.

Doctors must allow a certain length of time for symptoms to be happening, to rule out symptoms of a fever, such as flu, or an injury, like muscle strain. In the UK it usually takes a few days to get blood test results back, so even if you wake up unable to move and call the doctor right away, it is likely you will have been feeling unwell for a week or two by the time you get to see the doctor for the second time. Because of the chance that PMR symptoms can flare into giant cell arteritis while a patient is waiting for a diagnosis and not on medication, it is really important for you to be on the lookout for GCA symptoms such as a new severe headache, especially if it is accompanied by any visual disturbance such as blurring or interrupted vision, or jaw pain on chewing (more of this in the GCA section).

Aching of both shoulders (bilateral aching) and/or pelvic girdle aching

Your doctor will want to be satisfied your discomfort is on both sides of the body, that both your shoulders and/or both your hips are experiencing pain and stiffness. This is characteristic of PMR. They will ask questions to convince themselves that you have inflammatory pain, which is typically worse in the early hours of the morning, or during the second half of the night, worse when you are resting and is less bad if you move a little.

Like many people, before I fell ill with PMR, I had long since learned to live with aching shoulders. They have been a fact of life ever since office work became computer work. Most of us working in sedentary jobs are familiar with chronic tension in our shoulders and necks, reaching a crescendo by the end of the day, bringing on the classic "tension headache" on the journey home.

How is the pain of PMR different from this? My customary shoulder tension and ache was around my shoulder blades. The PMR pain on the other hand seemed to start right on the ridge of my shoulders and radiate up into my neck and down into my upper arms. Getting dressed, doing up my bra, brushing my hair were particularly painful. The bilateral aspect of this pain, i.e. that both sides of the body should be affected, is important in the classification of PMR. If it isn't on both sides, it is more than likely something else. It is unusual for the shoulders to be unaffected, but it can happen that the pain is felt first, or only, in the hip region. Another difference is that, with the tension ache, rotating the shoulders or shrugging them energetically to release the tension can often feel good. In PMR, trying to push through the pain doesn't help. Movement has to be gentle.

It wasn't until I started to really struggle getting up from my office chair that I realised the pain was spreading. I was feeling it deeper in my body, deep down inside the muscles, deep in my buttocks, and almost even deeper. I also knew instinctively that my actual joints, my shoulder and hip joints, that is, the bony bits, were absolutely fine. Their mobility was not impeded. It was the soft tissues around the joints causing so much rigidity. So much so it used to irritate me beyond reason when some innocent kind-hearted soul would ask "And how are your joints today?"

For some PMR sufferers who have the illness particularly severely, the pain is intense, like a Chinese burn, except you cannot kick your little brother to make it stop. It is more, far more, than feeling a bit achy.

We need to understand a little about the anatomy of the shoulders and hips, or more specifically, the shoulder girdle and pelvic girdle. The term *girdle* refers to the structure of connected bones, which in the case of the shoulder allows for movement in multiple directions, and in the case of the pelvis, protects the internal organs of the lower abdomen while providing a secure anchor for the legs. The shoulders and hips are often referred to in medicine as the *proximal joints*, the joints connecting our big limbs to our trunks. The big muscles are called the *proximal muscles*. They do the incredibly important job of keeping our body together and provide the motor engines for the joints that move our arms, legs and head.

Imaging, in the form of ultrasound, MRI, and CT-PET scans, is giving clinicians and researchers new insights into how the inflammation of PMR is affecting our bodies. In PMR the bones and muscles themselves are not inflamed, but the soft tissues around them may well be. Much of the pain we experience as muscle pain may actually be referred pain from these tissues.

Imaging may show up *tenosynovitis*, or inflammation in the synovial lining around tendons, especially of the biceps tendon at the shoulder. Another form of inflammation common in PMR is bursitis, or inflammation of the bursas, those sacs that contain fluid and provide a kind of cushion between bones and tendons in complex joints such as the shoulder, hips and spine. Bursitis at the shoulders and on the outer side of the hips are hallmark features.

And in some patients, these scans will show *synovitis*. The synovial membrane lines joints that have cavities, such as the shoulder and hip joints, and inflammation here can lead to a buildup of fluid and both in turn can lead to pain. For patients who have synovitis linked to their PMR, pain will be felt in the joints, particularly on moving. The challenge for doctors here is that joint synovitis is the key finding in rheumatoid arthritis, and even inflammation in the hallmark areas for PMR can be seen in rheumatoid as well. In some people, there is pain in the hands, which is also hard to differentiate from rheumatoid. In some cases, the distinction only becomes clearer with time, as the pattern of symptoms and signs evolves.

Finally, in the last few years several studies from around the world have used imaging to show that about 25% of people with PMR, without any of the cranial (head) symptoms of GCA, have evidence of underlying vasculitis, usually of the larger arteries[14]. This raises the possibility that, in these patients, PMR symptoms may partly be due to reduced blood flow to the muscles caused by underlying inflammation of the arteries. This is still an area of ongoing research and is not yet a proven explanation for PMR as a whole. However, this theory resonates with me; if the big muscles are hurting because they are short of oxygen and nutrients, then it stands to reason that they will feel awfully stiff and unwilling to move. It truly is a systemic illness and it's not surprising that it brings fatigue, sometimes weight loss, and a feeling of general unwellness.

The temporal artery biopsy for suspected cases of GCA, which takes away a small 'expendable' section of artery from just below the skin of the temple, is the closest we can get to definite evidence of what is going on deeper down in the body in GCA. Biopsy is not available for PMR, even if we would want it to be. We cannot very well open people up and check inside their shoulders and hips on a routine basis to work out what is going on.

That said, ultrasound can pick up the hallmark features of PMR at the shoulders and hips, although it's not that good at discriminating between PMR and rheumatoid. A team in Germany[15] recently found that MRI can show in great detail the characteristic and distinctive pattern of inflammation in the soft tissues around joints, but a research team in Australia has had even more remarkable results with CT-PET[16]. Here, a tiny amount of radioactive sugar called FDG-18 is taken up by inflamed cells, highlighting areas of inflammation, while the CT scan acts as a map to show exactly where these changes are in the body.

PET-CT can be particularly helpful because it shows the pattern of inflammation across the whole body in a single scan. It is this combination and distribution of findings, rather than one isolated feature, that makes the doctor more confident about the diagnosis[16]. Increasingly, for this reason, plus also because it can pick up GCA and other occasional PMR mimics like cancer and infection, PET-CT is regarded as the imaging gold standard for PMR diagnosis in the research world.

However, like it or not, PMR is unlikely to be very high on the priorities list for routine PET-CT for a long time to come (except for research), because it is expensive (at about £1000 per scan) and only generally available by specialist referral. Plus, the abnormal findings soon improve after steroids are started. At present, imaging such as ultrasound, MRI and PET-CT are usually only used in a selected portion of people referred to rheumatologists where it is not clear what is going on.

Morning stiffness

Ah, morning stiffness. This one makes me smile, and not in a good way. I felt stiff *all the time*. I'm not the only one. That phrase "morning stiffness" often raises a hollow laugh among groups of PMR sufferers. We're probably all familiar with the sensation of waking up feeling as though our limbs and back have turned into MDF during the night. In a healthy person, stretching like a cat will get everything moving again. Not so with polymyalgia rheumatica. People tell stories of having to be physically manhandled into a sitting position by a long-suffering partner.

At times, in the early hours of the morning, I would cry out in pain, half asleep, and my husband would patiently get out of bed, come round to my side, and turn me over. What must it be like for people on their own? I heard about one woman who tied a rope to rails on the foot of her bed so that she could haul herself up inch by inch like a mountain climber. Others have taken to sleeping in an armchair. It just shows how desperate people get.

A large proportion of PMRGCAuk members report they experience stiffness whenever they have been sitting or standing still for any length of time, at any time of the day. Drivers, on reaching their destination, have to lift their legs up with their hands to put them outside the car and plant their feet on the ground. In meetings, we have to get up and walk around to loosen ourselves up. Otherwise, we make an exhibition of ourselves when the meeting ends. Asking for a push-up from a colleague can be a bit embarrassing, and not very dignified.

One area of stiffness that has not received much attention yet from rheumatologists or researchers is the buttocks area. Sitting for any length of time, especially on a hard chair, can lead to intense pain and stiffness in the backside. Interestingly, the new research in Australia that I mentioned above has identified quite intense areas of inflammation around the buttocks, the rear of the pelvic girdle to be precise, which bears out what patients have been saying. It also reinforces the view that PMR is not just a localised condition, but affects the whole body, shoulders, hips, knees, thighs, neck and hands, and backside.

While doctors tend to make a clear distinction between pain and stiffness, for PMR sufferers they are two sides of the same coin[17]. They are the evil twins that stalk us, always together. They are the ropes that shackle us to the dragon's rock. The stiffness of PMR for me was more like a paralysis. However much I talked to my body and teased it, entreated it, implored it to move, it would not. And when the pain was bad, it was impossible to concentrate, to work, to get on with daily life. It went beyond any pain I had ever experienced in my muscles or joints before.

PMR makes people, literally, *dis-abled.*

The pain is associated with rigidity, and the stiffness – well, it ruddy well hurts. It is not like the almost pleasant stiffness and ache that comes into tired muscles after some intense physical activity, like walking up a mountain, or doing a day's gardening. It is not the kind of stiffness that melts away with a warm bath or a good massage. If only it did!

Elevated ESR

The ESR (Erythrocyte Sedimentation Rate) test is a blood test that measures the rate at which red blood cells settle in a blood sample within a period of one hour. Erythrocyte is the scientific term for a red blood cell. The rate of sedimentation of these cells in a sample of anticoagulated blood is an indicator of inflammation of the body. A substance called *fibrinogen*, also present in the blood, increases in quantity when there is inflammation present, and this causes the red blood cells to stick together, becoming heavier and falling to the bottom of the tube. A higher sedimentation rate is an indicator of inflammation. However, it is a bit of a blunt instrument.

While a normal ESR level in a healthy middle-aged adult might be around 20 to 30, a person with PMR or GCA might have a rate over 50 to 100. Yet if the ESR returns to normal, or towards normal, it does not necessarily mean that there is no disease present. Throughout my illness, my ESR rate never went above 50 (for this reason I was classified as atypical) and most of the time it was around 28 while I was on steroids. However, I was evidently and obviously ill. Plus, it can go up with other things wrong with us, such as kidney problems and anaemia, and it goes up as we get older and is higher in women than men.

Elevated CRP

The C-Reactive Protein test is a blood test that gives a measure of, yes, you guessed it, inflammation in the body. Cytokines are small protein molecules released by cells which act as messengers within the immune system. One category of cytokine is the interleukin (known as IL-1, IL-6 and so on). IL-6 is a little number that is released to stimulate the immune response. As it is the immune system going into battle that triggers inflammation in various parts of the body, the levels of IL-6 are a good indication of the levels of inflammation. IL-6 is an alarm system and CRP is produced in response and plays a part in cleaning up the molecular debris caused by cell death and breakdown. Its level rises rapidly in phases of acute inflammation, sometimes as much as 500-fold. Researchers have found levels of IL-6 and CRP are often higher in people with PMR than with late onset rheumatoid arthritis. Tests to measure IL-6 are expensive and not widely available, but the CRP test is cheap and available in all NHS hospitals.

Not everyone with PMR will have a raised ESR and/or CRP, but the majority do. So, if yours were normal before starting steroids that's another orange flag to ask to see a rheumatologist about your diagnosis.

The biochemistry of all these reactions and counterreactions going on, triggered by and modified by the immune system, is incredibly complicated and finely balanced. Not surprising if, sometimes, these tests turn out to be pretty unreliable when it comes to judging how a patient with PMR or GCA is progressing.

Whatever your ESR and CRP levels, make sure that your doctor has run a *full* set of laboratory blood tests before confirming the diagnosis.

Rapid response to steroids

Once you pick up your first prescription of prednisolone (or prednisone in the US) and take your first dose, you should feel remarkably better, sometimes within hours. In my own case, three hours after taking my first dose of 20mg, I felt a strange tingling all over my body and then jumped out of the chair and ran upstairs as though there was nothing wrong with me. Mine was a rather extreme reaction, and not everyone has the same experience.

At least a 70% improvement in symptoms should be felt within a week. You should be able to say that 70% of your pain and stiffness is relieved. Again, this shouldn't be used to clinch a diagnosis. It is a criterion for classifying PMR in general, not a criterion for diagnosis in specific cases. This is because almost any inflammatory illness will respond in the short term to steroids. Before the patient goes on steroids, many other possibilities need to be considered, such as different kinds of arthritis, infection, Parkinson's, and even various cancers. Also, a slower or lesser response might still be PMR, but it would be quite atypical and should raise alarm bells that something else might be going on. The reaction to steroids should also be sustained over time. If they stop working after a short while, this might call the initial diagnosis of PMR into question.

Diagnosis of PMR – primary or secondary care?

We can see that PMR is tricky to diagnose. It is largely a process of eliminating everything else. PMR is what you are left with, and a diagnosis of PMR will be supported by high ESR and CRP values in blood tests. Another issue is that many rheumatologists consider that PMR is being over-diagnosed by family doctors.

Vanessa worked with a team of researchers at Bristol Royal Infirmary who had established a polymyalgia rheumatica rapid access clinic in 2007 and monitored referrals for several years. Their aim was to increase the rate of early referrals to give them the chance to examine cases that would probably normally only be seen in primary care. They asked GPs to refer to them any suspected cases of PMR that fitted certain criteria – that is, with bilateral shoulder pain (both shoulders), increased acute phase response (elevated blood test results), and not yet on steroids. They aimed to see referred patients within two to three weeks.

After three years, the fascinating outcome of this experiment was that *only 55% of these patients turned out to have PMR*. The rest had a combination of late onset rheumatoid arthritis (LORA), some other shoulder problems, illnesses that could be viral, autoimmune, or even malignant (1 in 100), or GCA[18]. The team considered that having a rapid response PMR clinic can therefore screen out a lot of non-PMR cases that would otherwise be on steroids prescribed by GPs for months and months before getting a referral to a rheumatology clinic.

A new study from Ireland[19] demonstrates real-world outcomes of a dedicated fast-track polymyalgia rheumatica clinic. 39% of patients referred with suspected PMR had an alternative diagnosis for which a course of steroids was inappropriate. 55% of the non-PMR diagnoses were other inflammatory rheumatological conditions requiring follow-up. This work corroborates the earlier Bristol work and reinforces the idea that rheumatologists should see possible PMR patients, as most of the other things it could be, fall under the umbrella of rheumatological conditions.

Thousands of people may be on long-term steroid medication who do not need to be. Thus, although PMR is not really a life-threatening illness, there are many reasons why we need to improve diagnosis.

The recently published Guidelines of the French Society of Rheumatologists[20] for the diagnosis and treatment of PMR recommend rapid referral to rheumatology once PMR is suspected. In case of diagnostic doubt, ultrasound or PET imaging may be used to help. It would be nice to think that UK practice could follow the French example. I can be realistic and agree that, in today's NHS, this isn't likely to happen anytime soon.

In 2021, NHS England, in its wisdom, thrust a spanner into the works by commissioning a Getting It Right First Time document (GIRFT) on Rheumatology services in the NHS. It specifically states that PMR can generally be diagnosed and treated in primary care, i.e. by general practitioners[21]. The rationale for the GIRFT report was that most rheumatology services in the UK don't have the capacity to run PMR rapid access clinics, plus PMR is sadly still seen as a straightforward condition, easily dealt with in primary care. GPs are quietly advised to refer only the atypical or tricky cases to consultant rheumatologists at the local hospital. Rheumatologists thus never see most typical cases, and they don't get to include them in their research studies. One consequence of this is that research into PMR might be skewed by having an unrepresentative sample. PMR is an under-researched illness. If all suspected cases were referred, specialists would soon appreciate the extent of the problem and it might, just might, attract more research attention.

The GIRFT report was a disappointment at the time, but Vanessa and I are hopeful that a combination of education, lobbying and new research evidence will see some flexibility appearing in this position.

Putting anybody onto long-term steroid treatment carries risks to their health, so if we think of fast track PMR referral as a "stopping steroids" programme for people who turn out not to have PMR, the overall health benefits would be immense. So, in an ideal world, everyone with suspected PMR would be referred to a specialist for assessment. But we are not in an ideal world. Like it or not, it would entail enormous resource management problems for the NHS.

The latest UK and international recommendations, shortly to be published, will hold back from recommending referral for everybody, limiting it to atypical cases. These are not yet defined, but may include those with peripheral inflammatory arthritis, low inflammatory blood markers, age younger than 55, those suffering from significant steroid side effects, and cases where the patient flares or finds it impossible to reduce the steroids. If, as a result, GPs start consistently referring these patients, and rheumatologists accept the referrals, this will be a huge first step forward. Referral would also be appropriate if an alternative to prednisolone is a better option for people with complex pre-existing conditions, or certain risk factors complicate the prognosis. More on this later!

Here is the story of Val's experience of being diagnosed, or not diagnosed, with PMR. Rather unusually, her GP referred her at the beginning, but it didn't help much. It is a particularly messy case, but not untypical. I reproduce Val's story in her own words here just to give a flavour of how confusing and distressing it can be. You might recognise some things about it.

> *"I was 72 years old...having pains and stiffness in my shoulders and arms. Getting out of bed in the morning was torture as I was in so much pain that it made me cry with every move. It felt like flu, but I knew it wasn't. I went to see the GP who said, "I am almost 99% sure you have PMR, but I would like you to see a rheumatologist as I do not want to start you on steroids until we have a more concrete result."*

"I had to wait a couple of months before I got an appointment and was taking Co-codamol for the pain. The rheumatologist said that she was not sure if it was PMR or Fibromyalgia and she would take some blood tests etc. She then told me that as she was retiring, she would make an appointment for me to see the rheumatologist who was taking over from her, but this lady would not be able to see me for another six months, and in the interim, I should take pain killers.

"I went back to my GP and asked if I could have a second opinion, and she agreed, and asked if I had anyone in mind. I said that there was a neurologist in another hospital, and could I see her, if possible, if there was a chance it was fibromyalgia?

"The Neurologist confirmed to the GP that I do have PMR and that I should be taking steroids and be monitored regularly. Soon after this my GP told me that she was going to be on Maternity leave for six months, and one of the other doctors would take care of me.

"I started on 20mg per day. After a few hours, the pain disappeared and I became like a spring chicken, all stiffness gone. This other doctor did monitor me every 2 weeks for about 2 months, then he said that I should be thinking of reducing the pred, in order to come off it as soon as possible. Before taking the Pred, I was unable to lift my arms, this went when I started them, now I am finding it difficult to lift them again. I have been putting it down to the reduction of the Pred.

"The GP said that being on them for four years was a long time, and he was not sure if I really had PMR and, because of my age, it could be simply aches and pains as "this is what older people get", and the only way was to take pain

killers. Not being happy with this, I went to see one of the other doctors in the surgery, and she told me that perhaps I should see a rheumatologist at the local hospital, as the neurologist had discharged me for my own GP to be looking after me.

"When this rheumatologist told me that in his opinion I did not have PMR he said, "You do not get pain with it", although he prodded me on the shoulders and arms. He said with PMR you definitely do not get pain. He said he was also not sure, but it could be Fibromyalgia but again not so sure about that either. He told me to have some more blood tests taken and would see me again in May, I said if what you are telling me, that I am going to be in extreme pain, and finding that paracetamol does not work, could he recommend something else, his response was "go to a pain clinic, I don't deal with pain."

What strikes me as particularly awful about this sorry tale is that, in spite of having classic symptoms of PMR, and in spite of the GP being pretty confident about the diagnosis, Val had to go through weeks of pain, being shunted from pillar to post, before receiving effective treatment. This could be because GPs are not confident with PMR, and rheumatologists do not consider it particularly serious. Her doctors seemed to be playing a game of ping-pong between PMR and fibromyalgia. Medicine is so rigidly carved up into specialisms, and PMR, along with other autoimmune inflammatory illnesses, often falls through the gaps between them. Continuity of care was woefully lacking in this case.

Another sad aspect of Val's story is the way doctors continue to stereotype older people, and their symptoms as just part of getting old. And as for the rheumatologist who said that PMR isn't painful, well, that just makes me want to hit him round the head with a rheumatology textbook.

Early treatment of PMR – starting steroids

An overarching principle of treatment is to balance the benefits of controlling symptoms and disease activity against the potential harm of steroid-induced side effects. Finding the right dose to do this, particularly as the patient gets through the initial acute stage and starts to taper down, is a major preoccupation of treatment. Doctors are strongly urged in advisory documents to use the "minimum effective duration" of therapy and the "minimum effective dose".

But how to work out what that is?

The 2010 BSR (British Society of Rheumatology) guidelines for the treatment of PMR[2] suggest starting the patient off on 15mg of prednisolone per day, with a progressive tapering down once symptoms have stabilized. The 2015 ACR-EULAR (American and European Rheumatology) guidelines[3] recommend the starting dose be pitched somewhere between 12.5 and 25mg per day, depending on the patient's body size. I was in this working group, and I remember this criterion seemed rather rough and ready.

Newer PMR guidelines are more nuanced. The 2024 French guidelines recommend an initial weight-adjusted dose of 0.2 to 0.3 mg/kg/day adapted according to the patient's other health problems and disease activity[20], whilst the 2024 Norwegian Guidelines recommend an initial dose of 15 mg per day in most; up to 25 mg per day for those at increased risk of flare with low risk of developing steroid-related side effects, and between 10-15 mg daily for those at increased risk of developing steroid-related adverse effects[22].

After a couple of weeks on that starting dose, symptoms should be well under control, and the patient should be feeling much better. A key point is the four-week review after commencement of steroid therapy. At this point the doctor should discuss an individualised tapering scheme with the patient, with regular monitoring, involving blood tests and discussion of side effects. If the patient hasn't responded well to steroids in the early stages, this should trigger a reassessment of the diagnosis. It follows that the early weeks of treatment are also a period in which the doctor should make sure that the patient is receiving information and support to understand the condition and the treatment regime. Has this been your experience?

You will probably find your doctor very keen to get you down to about 12.5mg or 10mg a day pretty quickly, say, within the second month of your treatment, and to do this before your body gets too dependent on your starting dose. These steps down may be of 2.5mg at a time. It can be straightforward to get down from 15 to 12.5mg but take a little longer to make it down to 10. All the guidelines suggest that the aim of early tapering should be to get down to 10mg a day within four to eight weeks of starting treatment. For people starting on a higher dose, they recommend rapid tapering, whereas if the patient starts on a lower dose, such as 12.5mg a day, it might be acceptable to stay on the starting dose for longer. We talk much more about tapering in Chapter Four.

Patient perspectives

The PMRGCAuk helpline regularly takes calls from people newly diagnosed with PMR who are struggling to come to terms with the diagnosis and what it means for them. The most common concern voiced by these new patients is the fear of being on steroids for a long time. Some are worried their starting dose is so high and have not understood that it will drop over time. Many people want to avoid starting on them altogether and are looking for a viable alternative. They ask whether they can manage without taking the steroids, and whether paracetamol might be an adequate substitute. Paracetamol for most people is acceptable as a back-up pain relief. However, it doesn't deal with the inflammation of the disease and therefore doesn't work at all well for pain and stiffness due to PMR.

This tension between wanting to be free of symptoms and wanting to avoid side effects is a major challenge and a recurring theme in our experience. We will look at it in much more detail in Chapter Three, where we take a cold hard look at the risks posed by long-term steroid therapy.

Your doctor is likely to direct you to take all your tablets at once, early in the day. This is for several reasons. Firstly, because your symptoms may be worse in the mornings; secondly, prednisolone may have the effect of keeping you awake if taken later in the day, and also because this mimics the body's natural production of its own steroid hormone called cortisol, allowing your body to adjust more easily to the medication. Your doctor might instruct you to follow a low salt, high potassium, or high calcium diet. They should also prescribe or recommend a vitamin D supplement (with added calcium if you are not getting enough in your diet), to protect bone density. Follow these directions carefully and if possible, get a bone density scan.

There are social and economic factors that I hope your GP would consider when having the conversation with you about your treatment, and how your illness is impacting on you. You could be assessed not only on your physical condition but also consulted with about circumstantial factors such as those listed below. If they don't come up, help your GP by bringing up any that affect you:

- Are you in employment? What is the nature of your employment and how sympathetic and supportive is your employer likely to be?
- Are you a carer? If you were unable to continue caring because of PMR/GCA, what would the consequences be for the family?
- What is your current level of physical activity? How different is this from before you became ill?
- Do you already have weight/obesity issues? How much will you be affected if you gain more weight while on steroids?

- Do you have pre-existing chronic health issues, such as high blood pressure, familial hypercholesterolaemia, a history of cardiac problems, liver, kidney or gastric problems that the steroids will affect?
- Are you already frail? The French guidelines[20] mention that this should be considered. "Frailty" in these terms refers to pre-existing conditions of unintentional weight loss, fatigue, a low level of physical activity, muscular weakness and/or slow walking speed. If an older person presents without any of these factors, the French doctor may consider them "robust". One or two of these factors being present would signal someone who is "pre-frail", and three or more of them indicate frailty.
- How proactive are you likely to be in managing your condition yourself? Who else in your life needs to know about and understand PMR?

Granted, PMR is generally not life-threatening and people who start well have a fair prospect of recovery. But it is a serious illness and potentially grave because of the collateral damage it can do. Your GP should at least have the conversation that treats you holistically and as an individual. Also, informing patients of the risk and cardinal symptoms of GCA is paramount. It is amazing how many PMR patients have no idea. It's as though, having finally got a diagnosis, the GP breathes a sigh of relief, writes the prescription, and shows the patient the door.

A recent short piece in the Lancet Rheumatology journal put forward the case that PMR has been neglected by medics and researchers alike[23]. It hasn't been taken seriously enough in terms of developing new drug treatments. Prednisolone mops up the inflammation, but it won't modify the underlying disease. A new generation of biologic drugs is becoming available, but PMR is not currently seen as a sufficient priority to justify fast tracking the use of these high-cost therapies, leaving prednisolone as the mainstay of treatment on the NHS. This might have been just about acceptable in the past when it was generally believed that PMR was a self-limiting condition with a two-year timespan, and when other effective treatments did not exist. Now, there is clear evidence that around 25% of patients are on steroids for four years or longer. And there are alternatives out there. We will look at these more closely later.

Next up is the section on GCA. If you "only" have PMR, I recommend you read this section because up to one in ten people with PMR end up with a GCA diagnosis, so it's important to know about it, in case it's you!

Giant cell arteritis: identifying and diagnosing GCA

Giant cell arteritis is a vascular inflammatory disease affecting the arteries. Ever since GCA was first described in medical science, the major focus has been the arteries of the head, and particularly the temporal artery. Compared to the arteries deep in our bodies, the temporal arteries are relatively easy to see and even examine and logically linked to the headache traditionally the 'cardinal' symptom of GCA. Added to this is the real risk that, if the arteries of the eye become blocked by inflammation, a 'stroke in the eye' can occur, in turn leading to sight loss that is irreversible[24].

GCA and large vessel vasculitis

At some point around your diagnosis or a little later, you may hear your doctor or doctors dropping the term *large vessel vasculitis* into the conversation. This can be quite disconcerting, as it might give the impression you have another illness as well, or that the GCA diagnosis is in question, or the GCA has turned into something else.

Modern imaging techniques have shown what rheumatologists have long suspected: many cases of GCA also exhibit inflammation in the arteries of other parts of the body. The very large arteries in the chest cavity are crucially involved here – the aorta, the biggest artery in the body, and its main branches that feed blood into the neck, the head and the arms. Those with large vessel GCA tend to be on steroid medication for longer and have a greater need for steroid-sparing drugs. They also have a higher risk of aortic complications further down the line. This makes careful control of blood pressure important for these patients.

Vanessa gives an explanation here that should clear up any confusion or at least explain why the confusion exists. And it also helps to explain why your experience may be very different from that of another person with GCA.

Vanessa says: on GCA and large vessel vasculitis

There are many kinds of vasculitis, which are grouped into three subtypes: small-vessel, medium-vessel, and large-vessel. GCA is the most common large vessel vasculitis (LVV for short). There are other rarer kinds of vasculitis affecting the large vessels, like Takayasu's arteritis, ANCA-associated vasculitis and IgG4 disease, which have different clinical features and imaging findings to GCA, which is how we differentiate them.

GCA itself is divided into subtypes depending on symptoms, examination findings and imaging findings. If someone just has inflamed arteries around their head, typically the temporal arteries and arteries serving the eye and jaw muscles, then they tend to get head symptoms like sight loss, headache and jaw pain, and the temporal artery ultrasound or biopsy is more likely to be positive. These people are described as having cranial GCA or C-GCA.

If someone just has inflamed arteries in the chest cavity, neck and limbs (these are the very biggest arteries of the body, such as the aorta, carotids and axillary arteries), then they are described as having large vessel GCA (LV-GCA). This is confusing terminology because <u>all</u> GCA is large vessel GCA. It would be more precise to say VERY-large vessel GCA (I've just *made that up; no one actually calls it that!). In fact, some specialists prefer to call (very) large vessel GCA "extra-cranial" GCA, i.e. GCA outside the head area, just because of this confusion.*

Those with (very) large vessel GCA tend to have fewer head symptoms and are more likely to have PMR and "constitutional symptoms" like night sweats, low-grade fever, weight loss and anaemia on blood tests. Their inflamed blood vessels may show up on axillary artery ultrasound, or on CT, MRI or CT-PET scans of their torso and neck. When someone has features of both cranial and large vessel GCA, then we say they have mixed GCA.

As a very rough guide, about 50% of people with GCA just have cranial GCA, about 20% just have large vessel GCA (LV-GCA), and about 30% have mixed GCA. So about 50% of people have LV-GCA as part of their GCA. The different GCA subtypes can happen from the outset, or people may get one, then the other, alone or together.

---- x ----

Here's the bottom line. If you have GCA and are told you have large vessel vasculitis, you probably have the variant affecting about 50% of people with GCA, where the very biggest arteries of the body are affected. You do not have two separate conditions.

Signs and symptoms

As we have learned, there is quite a cluster or spectrum of sub-types of GCA. The recognition that GCA can include a whole range of arteries around the head and body makes sense of it being a systemic disease affecting the whole person, giving rise to no end of signs and symptoms.

Here's a list, collated from many studies in patients in whom GCA was already suspected[25,26].

• Headache	72%
• Headache in the temple	66%
• Temporal artery abnormality	53%
• Loss of appetite	40%
• Weight loss	39%
• Scalp tenderness	39%
• Jaw claudication	38%
• Visual disturbance	34%
• PMR	33%
• Fever	27%
• Aching joints	25%
• Arm or leg claudication	20%
• Permanent loss of vision	22%
• Previous PMR	19%
• Transient loss of vision	11%
• Double vision	7%
• Stroke	3%

Other recognised symptoms of GCA include:

- Pain in the back of the neck
- Shoulder or hip girdle stiffness without clear PMR diagnosis
- Cough (often dry and persistent)
- Sore throat or throat discomfort
- Facial pain (can mimic dental or sinus problems)
- Hearing loss or tinnitus
- Dizziness or vertigo
- Asymmetrical pulses or blood pressure differences between arms
- Chest or back pain (might suggest aortic involvement)
- Tongue claudication (tongue pain when speaking/eating)
- Scalp or tongue infarction or tissue damage (rare but highly specific for GCA)

As in PMR, most people have a raised CRP and or ESR, but not all, and about half are anaemic. Here are the percentages:

• Raised CRP and/or ESR	96%
• Raised CRP	87%
• Raised ESR	83%
• Anaemia	56%

This is one heck of a mixed bag, both for patients and doctors, and it is salutary to read it and mentally check all those symptoms that could easily be taken as a sign of something else, especially if you are older and have one or more chronic conditions already. Also, it's really striking that 3 out of 10 people don't have the headache considered the cardinal symptom of GCA.

Suppose a man, let us call him Cliff, is experiencing pain in his jaw when he tries to chew his food. His first thought is his dentures are playing up. Cliff hates going to the dentist, but eventually he plucks up courage. Again, the dentist may not be looking in the right place. It takes a bit of joined-up thinking for a dentist, an ophthalmologist or even a GP to start suspecting GCA.

Imagine a 76-year-old woman called Mary starts to experience blurry vision, as well as headaches. Perhaps she has noticed her scalp feels tender sometimes. Mary goes to the GP and says that her sight seems a bit blurry. The doctor is likely to suspect, say, glaucoma, because this is far more common than GCA. If Mary remembers to mention the headaches, the doctor will suggest she goes to the optician, or the ophthalmologist, to have her sight checked out. Meanwhile perhaps she could take paracetamol for the headaches. Mary completely omits to mention the occasional tender scalp. Why should she remember it, as it does not seem to have anything to do with the blurriness? She makes an appointment to have her eyes tested. The ophthalmologist, maybe a week or ten days later, checks out her eyes. There may be some signs of glaucoma developing. However, the eye specialist will not see any evidence of the storm brewing up in Mary's arteries. Why not? Because the problem is in the arteries supplying the eye and has not yet caused any damage in the actual eyes at all.

Here's the story of Jeff in the US, bringing this to life:

> *"I had PMR unknowingly for several months before the GCA symptoms started. At that time, I didn't know anything about PMR and GCA, and I blamed the symptoms on other things, such as aging and a sinus infection. I went to two doctors because of my symptoms, an orthopaedist and an ear, nose, and throat doctor, and neither one diagnosed the PMR or GCA.*
>
> *"The first symptom I had of GCA was a low-grade fever. Initially it lasted about 2 or 3 hours a day, but it lasted longer and longer and increased in temperature over time. The next symptom was pain in my cheekbones. I sleep on my side, and the pressure of the pillow against my cheekbones was very uncomfortable. Then jaw claudication started. My jaw muscles would become very tired while I was eating, and I started to dread meals. I wear glasses, and I started having a lot of pain around my ears where the earpieces of my glasses touched my ears. I also had some tenderness in my scalp. Occasionally the air moving from a ceiling fan would cause pain on my scalp. I never had any headaches from the GCA.*
>
> *"The combination of PMR and GCA made it difficult to sleep, I took a lot of acetaminophen (paracetamol) during that time, which helped some. Sometimes when I was in bed at night, I would debate with myself about whether it would be worth the pain to turn over to get into a more comfortable position.*
>
> *"The symptom that finally resulted in my diagnosis was vision problems in my left eye. One night I got up to use the*

> *restroom, and suddenly all I could see in my left eye was a solid grey curtain. It only lasted for a few seconds. I thought I might have had a stroke, so I went to the emergency room. While there I had several more episodes of vision disturbances in my left eye. During those episodes some colors would disappear, and other colors would spread out. It was like looking at an impressionist painting. I was diagnosed with GCA and admitted. I was there for 3 days and received an IV each day of methylprednisolone. My vision was saved by that treatment along with the subsequent prednisone and Actemra (tocilizumab)."*

I'm so grateful to Jeff for sharing this story because it's such a beautiful example of how GCA doesn't play ball with the doctors. It's tricky because the average GP may only see a case of GCA once every three years or so. Some GPs have never seen one.

Doctors would use the term *amaurosis fugax* to describe Jeff's visual symptoms. This combines the Ancient Greek *amaurosis*, meaning a darkening or loss of vision, with the Latin *fugax*, meaning fleeting or transient, to describe a brief, temporary episode of visual loss. It's a symptom which really shouldn't be ignored, because 30-50% will go on to develop permanent visual loss if not treated promptly with steroids.

Jeff was lucky he took himself to the ER in time.

Improving diagnosis

When a doctor suspects GCA, they face a difficult balance: delaying steroid treatment risks irreversible sight loss, sometimes within hours, but starting steroids may make the diagnosis harder to confirm later. And it is important to be confident about the diagnosis of GCA, because the steroids needed can cause lots of side effects. It is a serious business to put a patient on steroids knowing they will potentially be on these drugs for two or three years, or even longer. The difficulty is that not all GCA cases are straight forward to diagnose. No single symptom, physical abnormality, or blood test tells the doctor you have GCA. Like PMR (remember the Magnificent Seven?), you need a combination of these for the doctor to be suspicious, and the more you have, the higher the chance you have GCA. In a similar vein, even if one of the usual features is missing, such as raised inflammatory markers or a Northern European background, GCA can still occur.

A GCA probability score (GCAPS for short, pronounced "G-CAPS"), based on all these features, has been developed by Professor Dasgupta and his team at Southend Hospital[27]. It may help your doctor with this conundrum. Quite a few rheumatology units across the UK have put this probability scoring system to the test over a few years and shown that it is pretty reliable for filtering out those patients who are less likely to have GCA. Using the GCAPS, a 55-year-old with a headache and no other features on this list plus a normal CRP and ESR has a very low probability of GCA and almost certainly has a headache for another reason.

Conversely, a 70-year-old with a headache, jaw pain on chewing, PMR symptoms, weight loss, fever and a raised CRP (if bloods have been done) is much more likely to have GCA. The doctor won't hang about before starting them on steroids to protect them from losing their sight (because the risk of starting steroids is less than the risk of them potentially having untreated GCA). However, even this 70-year-old might have something else going on, so to confirm the diagnosis of GCA, a specific GCA test is recommended in all people where GCA is suspected.

A biopsy of the temporal artery at the side of the forehead was for many years the standard way to do this. A positive biopsy would ideally contain one of those giant cells. Although it's generally low risk, it's still an invasive procedure. And for everyone it's really good news that the biopsy is rapidly being superseded by more modern imaging techniques, such as ultrasound and CT-PET scanning. In many hospitals, ultrasound scanning is now the first line of testing for GCA.

There have been more innovations and changes in GCA diagnosis over the last ten years, especially in Europe and the UK. A ground-breaking fast-track pathway was pioneered by Professor Wolfgang Schmidt in Berlin in the late 1990s, which became a model for similar initiatives around the world. The first highly influential pathway in the UK was set up in Southend by Professor Dasgupta in 2012[28] and similar pathways have sprung up widely since. Basically, a well-functioning fast-track pathway provides a GP, ophthalmologist or other hospital doctor who is concerned that a patient may have GCA, with an assurance that the patient will be seen urgently by a rheumatologist ideally within 3 days. The doctor can then start the patient off on a high dose of steroids as an emergency measure to prevent sight loss, without fearing that all the features of the disease will disappear in the time between the referral and the consultation at the hospital. If the patient turns out not to have GCA after all, the steroids can be stopped quickly without a long taper, because physical dependence hasn't yet been established. Proving that a fast-track pathway could improve diagnosis, and in fact, save money at the same time was a pivotal moment for the diagnosis and treatment of GCA.

At around the same time, campaigning by PMRGCAuk led to sight loss due to undiagnosed GCA being classified as an 'untoward' event and recorded on a monthly British register of sight loss. This meant hospitals had an external incentive to put in place changes to speed up access to specialists.

The Southend team first got agreement from all the GPs in their area that any suspected cases of GCA would be reported to them immediately. In return, they provided a special emergency call service, and 80% of people were seen within 24 hours. Within two years, the rate of sight loss fell from 37% to 9%.

We now have plenty of data, e.g. from a Norwegian study[29] and a study Vanessa carried out on her fast-track pathway in Luton, showing sight loss rates have reduced to around 10%. Getting below this towards zero is very tough, because most people who lose sight do so before they see any doctor. They might be the sort of people who don't want to bother the doctor with something like a headache, or they may have early dementia, or be unwell with other conditions. This is why it's so important for members of the public to be aware of GCA, especially those who have, or have had PMR, where the risk is higher. If you know about GCA, you can spot tell-tale signs and symptoms in yourself or those close to you and get help in good time.

At least half of NHS trusts in England and Wales are now trying to implement and maintain fast-tracks. This is real progress, because it needs dedicated resources, organization and effective communications, and ten years ago we couldn't have assumed these would be forthcoming for a condition like GCA (uncommon, old people, etc.).

Of course, if there is no local fast-track pathway or helpful rheumatologist or ophthalmologist, then the GP will need to start treating the case themselves. Steroids have to be got into those arteries to protect Cliff or Mary's sight, and the case can't wait for the hospital appointments system to catch up.

As well as reducing sight loss, introducing a fast-track pathway in an area improves the education of the referrers, and GPs become more sensitised to GCA symptoms. If the pathway is working, patients get seen within 1-3 days, blood tests can be taken quickly, the patient can be seen by a rheumatologist and have ultrasound scanning if necessary. They are then much more likely to end up with a secure diagnosis early on (one where the doctor is really confident that they do or don't have GCA).

Remarkably, the Southend pilot was able to demonstrate that the fast-track pathway was actually less expensive than the hit-and-miss approach that was there before.

The most surprising thing to me was learning that, consistently, up to three out of four people referred along fast-track pathways across the world turn out *not* to have GCA. For example, an Australian study reported that out of 137 people seen on the pathway, only 45 were confirmed with a GCA diagnosis. This is massively important, because it means these patients can immediately stop the steroids they are taking (to prevent GCA-related sight loss), without any need for tapering. In this sense the fast-track pathway is a stopping steroids service as well as a "stopping sight loss" service, something I hadn't really thought of.

Those negative diagnoses of GCA are as significant to the patients as the positive ones. These patients are the ones who got away. They may never think about GCA again, they will certainly never read this book, but it's good to know their lives have been improved by these advances in diagnosis because they haven't had to take long term steroids for a condition they never had. Furthermore, being able to rule in and rule out GCA quickly saves a huge number of unnecessary biopsies.

The reason fast-track is so important for rheumatologists is that, as soon as a GP prescribes steroids to protect the patient and the patient starts taking them, the clock starts ticking. Those elusive giant cells start disappearing and the tell-tale thickening of the artery walls reduces. If seen fast enough, a rheumatologist can often see whether a patient has GCA by just looking at them. The temporal artery appears knotty and swollen and feels sore when pressed. The technical term is *indurated* – hardened. An indurated temporal artery with rapid response to steroids is a very specific sign of GCA.

If there's a time lapse between starting steroids and being seen, four things happen to someone with GCA. The patient starts to feel better and the brain starts to forget what the symptoms were really like. Those knotty temporal arteries become less tender and swollen. The blood CRP count goes down, and the ultrasound scan is much more likely to be negative. CRP can drop to normal within a very few days, so it's vital to have bloods done as soon as possible after steroids are started. They should really be done on the same day. With every passing day, it becomes harder to see the tell-tale thickening on the scan. So clearly, getting the blood tests done and that ultrasound scan as quickly as possible is of the essence in best practice GCA diagnosis.

We now need a closer look at what ultrasound is all about. Before we do though, we need to say again that ultrasound scanning for GCA has become much more established in the UK and Europe than it is in the USA. If you're in the States or Canada, it's still more likely you will have a temporal artery biopsy, which we'll look at in more detail later in this chapter.

Ultrasound

Years ago, in patient groups, we had an impression that finding one or more giant cells in a sample of temporal artery under the microscope was the Holy Grail of GCA diagnosis. Nowadays, the presence of a characteristic halo pattern on an ultrasound scan image in a person with GCA symptoms has superseded the need to look for those giant cells. Put simply, the halo is the new giant cell. Paradoxically, the halo shows up as black on the image. It gives away the presence of swelling and inflammation in the artery wall, caused by the increased water content. The higher this water content, the blacker the halo shows on the scan.

In the scan of a healthy artery, the cross-section of the artery wall shows as an inner white line, and an outer white line, with a thin central black portion. The blood passing through the artery shows up on the scan as a reddish-yellowish area (because it's moving it creates a Doppler effect and therefore doesn't show up as black).

In a person sick with GCA, the whole artery wall appears as "off-black" and thicker, resembling a ring doughnut we talked about in the introduction. This is the halo. The more florid the halo, the more it is associated with sight loss in the patient. This is because the scanned temporal arteries often reflect what is happening to the arteries serving the eye. The eye arteries are hidden behind the eye and can't easily be scanned directly. As the halo gets thicker, the blood flow becomes totally inadequate to supply the eye and can thus lead to blindness: "a stroke in the eye."

Vanessa has some interesting things to say about rheumatologists learning about the potential of ultrasound for GCA diagnosis. It's actually quite challenging for rheumatology departments to set up ultrasound driven GCA fast-track pathways, because it takes several years to train staff, and at present, rheumatology trainees don't have any time set aside in their training to learn it, so they have to go the extra mile to learn, doing it in their study time or spare time, as Vanessa did. Temporal artery scanning is not part of an ultrasonographer's usual training. Not all rheumatology departments have ultrasound machines and Trusts are often not keen to spend the money, even if someone is keen to learn.

The other challenge is the need for the whole process to be done rapidly (ideally within three days) because the clock starts ticking as soon as the person starts to take steroids, and tests for GCA go negative quickly with steroid treatment. With each day of steroid treatment, it will become increasingly likely they won't find any artery wall inflammation, because the steroids have melted it away. This is why fast-track pathways are so important.

Vanessa says: on ultrasound:

When I started learning how to do ultrasound scanning for suspected GCA, there was no formal training structure and no training time given. The best course was in Norway, so I went over there, and also visited Professor Dasgupta in Southend.

In order to get practice and learn more about what the temporal artery looked like via ultrasound, I would do it in my lunch hour, with obliging patients who were going to have a biopsy. I couldn't use the scans to make decisions about patient care, but I could compare the results I was getting with the ultrasound to the results coming from the biopsies.

After the end of a year, I did an audit and was able to show that I would be able to use ultrasound to diagnose GCA.

It worked like this:

In patients where I figured there was a low probability of them actually having GCA, a negative ultrasound scan could rule out GCA. All my positive ultrasound scans were coming through with positive biopsies, so that was a pretty strong argument for using ultrasound to confirm a diagnosis without a biopsy in those cases where I was confident of GCA.

But in the middle, between the low probability patients and the clear positives, there were the cases where the ultrasound wasn't definitive, and those cases still needed a second test such as a biopsy. In the second year, we dramatically reduced the biopsy rate. With each subsequent year, our biopsy rate as a proportion of our suspected GCA patients has fallen further, because we have worked hard to see people quickly, we have become more experienced in ultrasound, and we got funding for a better ultrasound machine for our unit. Many people used to be treated just on the basis of their 'story' of their symptoms, and their response to steroids and I suspect people were treated for GCA who didn't have the condition, because doctors wanted to be cautious and didn't want to miss GCA and cause blindness. Our fast-track pathway with ultrasound scanning has completely changed things. Now almost all our patients have a secure diagnosis of GCA (usually confirmed on ultrasound, or with biopsy or other imaging). We have become more confident to withdraw steroids quickly in everyone else, so they are not on steroids unnecessarily. The fast-track stays open to them if symptoms come back and their GP is worried. Having a secure diagnosis is also important for access to the newer high-cost drugs we have for GCA (more on this later).

In recent years, rheumatology units around the UK have been setting up similar fast-track pathways. It's a challenging process and can't be done overnight. Progress is slower than we might like but going in the right direction.

---- x ----

If you are going to have an ultrasound scan for suspected GCA, it will take a little while, because all three segments of the temporal artery are looked at on both sides of the head. Also, the axillary arteries should be looked at; 8 segments in total:

- The common superficial temporal artery (just in front of the ear)
- The frontal branch – rising up over the eyebrow
- The parietal branch – going up into the hair.
- The axillary artery – best seen in the arm pit, sometimes up onto the upper chest.
- Then all are repeated on the other side.

Sometimes, other arteries will be scanned if the 8-segment scan is negative. Your rheumatologist may do the scan themselves or send you to a specially trained vascular ultrasound technician or radiologist. If, of course, there is one at your hospital. If you prefer, come in a thin strapped vest top, so the scanner can easily get to your arm pits without you completely undressing, and be prepared to have ultrasound gel around your temples and armpits.

Temporal Artery Biopsy

I was a little shocked to discover that some hospitals or healthcare procurement authorities are dragging their feet on ultrasound scanning because doing biopsies earns them more money. Yes. As a surgical procedure it carries a higher cost or value than an imaging session. So, although ultrasound equipment is much more widespread than ten years ago, it's still common for a patient to be told they need a biopsy. Don't hesitate if this is the case with you. It's still a good test for GCA. It's just that ultrasound is a more convenient first test, when it's available, because a much wider range of arteries can be scanned, it has no risks and can be repeated if needed.

Before surgery, you can eat, drink and take medications normally. For example, if you normally take warfarin or a DOAC (direct oral anti-coagulant), you do not have to stop taking it. The procedure usually takes place in the operating theatre, under local anaesthetic. You need to lie still for 30 to 45 minutes. The surgeon makes an incision in your temple and removes a small section of artery. This is usually only 2cm, or just under an inch, in length. The wound is about 3-4 cm long and, normally, absorbable sutures (stitches) are used. The biopsy then goes for examination under a microscope. You will be able to go home while waiting for the results to come through.

You will have a small dressing to cover the wound on your temple. There may be a small amount of pain for a short time after the anaesthetic wears off. Taking simple painkillers like paracetamol can help with this. You will need to continue taking the daily steroid dose as advised until your follow-up appointment. You can wash your hair carefully once advised it is safe to do so.

Every operation, no matter how big or small, carries a possible risk. However, the risks associated with temporal artery biopsy are very small. It is a safe procedure, but the *possible* complications are:

a. Post-operative infection – look out for redness which progressively increases in size, or a continuous discharge.
b. Increased inflammation and delayed wound healing – temporary redness and swelling to the temple area.
c. Bleeding – during the operation and perhaps until the evening of procedure. If you are on aspirin or warfarin, the risk of bleeding is greater.
d. A scar – this is often concealed in the hairline.

Very rarely, serious complications such as damage to nearby nerves causing forehead weakness or poor wound healing are reported, but Vanessa has not seen these in her practice.

Discuss these risks with the rheumatologist and/or the surgeon before you have the procedure.

It can be quite confusing for the patient, who is feeling unwell anyway so not in the best frame of mind, to discover that, although they have undergone this surgical examination and the biopsy has turned out to be negative, the doctors still are pretty convinced they have GCA. If this happens to you, you could be forgiven for wondering what the point of the biopsy was in the first place. In fact, few patients are informed that a third to a half the biopsy samples taken are thought to be negative because the person's GCA is affecting arteries other than the temporal arteries, or the sample was not long enough to 'catch' the typical inflammation seen in GCA. So up to half of biopsies may be false negatives, where the consultant is certain of the GCA diagnosis despite the negative biopsy result. You also have to be aware it isn't a treatment in itself. In fact, if I knew someone who was facing a biopsy, I would suggest they ask their consultant the question, "What if the biopsy comes back negative? Will you still think that I have GCA? Is biopsy the best test for me here?" Vanessa explains below how she would answer this question.

Vanessa says: on temporal artery biopsy

The biopsy result shifts the probability of GCA. A positive result is helpful because the doctor and the patient know what's wrong and can stay firm and confident with the plan for GCA treatment even when things don't go exactly as predicted. It also helps the doctor to get high-cost drugs such as tocilizumab if needed, as everyone believes the person has GCA. It also makes the doctor feel more comfortable about that person taking on the risk of tocilizumab because they will reap the benefit.

A negative result means the probability is lower but does not rule it out completely because of the false negative rate. Then the probability of GCA based on the person's symptoms, signs and blood tests comes into play. If they are very suggestive of GCA and other tests haven't flagged any other clear cause, I will make a "clinical diagnosis" of GCA. But I can't be certain they have GCA, so if things are not going as expected, I'll have a lower threshold for looking for other causes for the symptoms. However, if the person's symptoms are not so suggestive of GCA, then a negative biopsy will push down the probability of GCA low enough for me to advise the person to stop the steroids and for us to watch what happens.

I usually use temporal artery biopsy as a follow-up test after ultrasound when the clinical features and imaging have not clearly confirmed or excluded GCA. So, the ultrasound result is also feeding into the probability.

In someone with clinical features that suggest mainly large vessel GCA, imaging tests like CT-PET, CT or MRI may be more appropriate than a biopsy because they can look at larger blood vessels deeper in the body, including the aorta. PET-CT scans are particularly useful because they show how actively inflamed tissues are.

Any of these tests can be useful down the line if someone's GCA is not well controlled but the most likely time for them to be positive is at diagnosis.

---- x ----

Scanning the eye?

At this point, you may be wondering why there aren't better tests for directly imaging the arteries of the eye, seeing as after all this is where the brewing storm is of most danger. You might have heard of Optical Coherence Tomography (OCT) because it is available at many high-street opticians. It is a type of imaging of the eye giving a lot of information about the condition of the retina, and the blood supply to it. But OCT picks up the consequences, i.e., the damage caused by GCA, it does not pick up the storm itself. When used by an ophthalmologist (a doctor specialising in eyes), OCT can help identify eye changes caused by GCA as part of urgent specialist assessment, although it's not a test used on its own for GCA diagnosis. In contrast, high-street opticians can recognise suspicious changes on OCT, but they are not trained to interpret the findings like an ophthalmologist. In short, OCT cannot rule out GCA and should not be relied on as a screening test at the opticians.

Newer OCT that can map really, really tiny blood vessels and also trans-orbital ultrasound using very high frequency equipment are still mostly just used in research but may represent the future of imaging in GCA.

Early treatment of GCA

The standard treatment for GCA is to give the patient high dose steroids, generally prednisolone, to control the symptoms. If the patient has been admitted as an emergency, the first doses may be intravenous. A standard starting dose is 40-60mg. Much, much higher than the starting dose for PMR, because in the acute phase it is vital to shrink the swelling in the walls of the artery clogging up the blood flow, particularly to the eye and optic nerve. The steroids force the inflamed artery walls to shrink. Prednisolone is the drug of choice because it works. NSAIDs, or non-steroidal anti-inflammatory drugs, such as ibuprofen, do not have the same effect and you cannot control GCA with them. Once the symptoms are well under control, doctors will want to start reducing the dose as soon and as quickly as possible.

There is a good deal of debate and speculation about the optimum way of tapering steroids down from this initial high dose, and we dedicate Chapter Four to this. The trick is to keep on top of the symptoms and simultaneously reduce the medication as much as possible, since steroids are very powerful drugs that have other effects on the body. A patient on steroids will hopefully feel very much better very quickly.

If you have been diagnosed with GCA, it is tempting, after the steroids have kicked in and you are feeling much better, to think, "OK, that's sorted." The effect of steroids can literally seem like a miracle. You will think the dragon has slunk, beaten, into his lair. Nevertheless, you need to understand and accept you have a serious illness. The prednisolone does not cure it – but it does make it possible to live a reasonably normal life with GCA. Reducing the dosage too quickly will result in a flare of symptoms. It is important for patients and doctors to understand this and work together in the early weeks to learn how the disease is behaving in the individual, and how the medication is working. Keeping a log of symptoms is a good idea.

Remission?

This is as good a point as any to mention that there can sometimes be confusion around the term "remission". We lay people often understand it to be the complete absence of the disease. But doctors often say you are in remission when you are on steroids and your symptoms are under control. They are aiming for "clinical remission", i.e. suppression of the disease symptoms at the lowest possible effective dosage of medication. It doesn't feel like remission to you because you know if you don't take your meds, you will flare straight away. When your doctor talks about you being in remission, it might be worth checking which kind of remission they are talking about – remission on treatment, or complete drug-free remission.

In conclusion

In all probability you have grabbed a copy of this book after getting a diagnosis. So, the chapter you've just read might seem like shutting the stable door after the horse has bolted. But hopefully you'll have a clearer perspective now on why things happened for you the way they did. If you have PMR, then it is very useful for you to know about GCA and how it might develop, because a small minority of people with PMR do go on to be diagnosed with GCA, either whilst they are tapering their steroid, or after stopping. Experiences of both illnesses in the early stages can be quite different, and yet it's important for people to be aware of them. We need to get to the point where people are no longer taken utterly by surprise when they are diagnosed with PMR or GCA. These diseases are not rare. Talk about your experiences and your condition with family and friends. Society needs to know about it.

We have seen that GCA and PMR are closely related. However, the vast majority of PMR cases are diagnosed and treated in primary care by GPs, whereas GCA is viewed as a medical emergency and the diagnosis has to be made, or confirmed, clinically within a rheumatology department. Perhaps by the next edition of this book, most rheumatology departments will have a fast-track pathway for GCA. It would be marvellous if PMR were treated in the same way. It would mean rheumatologists would see and treat a wider range of PMR patients, and they could then be included in research studies.

I am not holding my breath, but we can hope and campaign for a wider range of PMR cases to be dealt with in secondary care, so rheumatologists and researchers will have more knowledge about the variations between patients and the different behaviour of these diseases.

3 Steroids

When I started on steroids, I went within hours from hobbling with a walking stick to running up the stairs. It felt like a miracle. People who have not experienced PMR might struggle to understand what "muscle pain all over the place" really is like. For me, the stiffness was of a completely different order from any kind of stiffness I had ever experienced before, including after running the London marathon. Then, if I mustered all my will, I could make my body move. The stiffness of PMR was more like a paralysis. However much I talked to my body and teased it, entreated it, implored it to move, it would not. The pain went beyond any pain I had ever experienced in my muscles or joints before. With this level of pain, it is impossible to concentrate, to work, to get on with daily life. PMR makes people literally dis-abled. The steroids give me my life back. But at a cost.

Just one dose of 20mg worked a miracle for me. GCA patients have told me that they had similar experiences with prednisolone. I liked Oxfordboy2's description in an email:

> *"At diagnosis my GP on hospital advice started me on 40mg prednisolone. Within two hours I was a new man, all symptoms disappeared. The pred made me very hyper on the top dose but that reduced as I tapered down. Such a shame pred comes with side effects because I would give anything to feel that good all the time."*

In this chapter we are going to take a long hard look at prednisolone and its effects on the body, in the short and long terms. From the initial high doses, where we can imagine the pred damping down the fiery head of the dragon, and subduing it, to the long process of weaning off the medication, prednisolone, a remarkably potent drug, is working not only on the inflammation but on our whole body too. This chapter will give insight into why it sometimes might seem that doctors are more preoccupied than anything else with getting you off pred. And why so many patients have a love-hate relationship with it.

For both of us, this chapter and the next have been the most difficult to write, because we have to give adequate attention to all these risks, but we don't want to be alarmist and make you expect a difficult time of it. Your doctor will perhaps have given you a schedule for reducing your steroid dose over time. This will assume that everything will go smoothly and you'll be able to reduce, hopefully to zero, without incident. If you read this chapter, you will be well-prepared if your experience turns out not to be so straightforward. Forewarned is forearmed. When patients get together, whether online or in person, there is at least as much talk about life on prednisolone, and getting off it, as there is about PMR and GCA.

Vanessa says: on prednisolone

Your doctors are aiming to support you to be the healthiest version of yourself, both now and in the future. Our plan for each person is to find that balance between the lowest level of symptoms and the lowest level of side effects from the medication for each person. We are thinking about your day-to-day symptoms and challenges, but also about any other health problems you have and about any health problems you may get in the future as a result of the treatment choices that are made today. I call this the "Goldilocks amount" of steroid - not too much, which increases risks from steroids, and not too little, which allows the disease to cause harm.

---- *x* ----

The ideal would be to know the Goldilocks amount of steroid for everyone, just the right amount to control the disease, not too much, at each point along the course of the disease. But this is often challenging, as there are several potential complications you and your doctor may be considering that might affect your taper. Plus, when it comes to tapering, the two of you are dealing much of the time in degrees of risk (probability of something happening), not in certainties. As well as the level of risk, another thing to be factored into the decision is your attitude to risk. In other words, how important it is to you to avoid risk (of flaring or of steroid side effects)?

What do steroids do?

The scientists (Kendall, Hench and Reichstein) who won Nobel prizes in 1950 for discovering cortisol as a natural anti-inflammatory product of the adrenal glands, revolutionised the treatment of inflammatory diseases. Synthetic versions of cortisol, prednisolone, or prednisone, soon became standard treatment for GCA and PMR. And thus it has remained for more than 70 years. Prednisolone is more commonly used in the UK and most of Europe, while prednisone is more common in North America. Essentially, they work in the same way.

Pred works by mimicking the natural product cortisol in the body, when the immune system of a patient is out of balance, and is over-producing cytokines, which are inflammatory substances in the bloodstream. Steroids dampen this process down, very effectively, and usually quite quickly. However, they don't deal with the underlying disorder that is causing the inflammation, which is why symptoms may return, and why it may be difficult to come off the drug. It takes time for the body to heal itself.

Whether you have GCA or PMR or both, once you've got over the brutal acute phase of feeling absolutely awful, once your symptoms have come under control and there is no longer an immediate risk to your sight, you will find your doctors seem terribly keen to get you off the steroids as soon as possible. This might seem paradoxical, seeing as our glucocorticoid chum, prednisolone (or prednisone) is doing such a good job. However, doctors are trained to approach it with caution because steroids, basically, are toxic.

All drugs are toxic in one way or another. If we take too much of anything, it will make us sick. In the case of pred, the damage can be creeping and cumulative. Even relatively small doses, taken over a long period, may damage our tissues and internal organs to some degree. In the case of PMR and GCA, it's the price we pay for being on top of our disease symptoms.

Starting doses and tapering

A typical starting dose for a person with a diagnosis of PMR is between 15 and 20mg of prednisolone per day. The starting dose for GCA is much higher. The British Society of Rheumatology Guidelines recommend 40-60mg per day, with 60mg for those with concerning eye symptoms or jaw claudication and 40mg for everyone else.

It is typical to maintain the starting dose for about two to four weeks, until acute signs and symptoms have resolved. I have a mental image of this initial drenching in steroids as a big bucket of water chucked at the head of the dragon, scaring him back into his lair, down but not out. The doctor should be keen to see a clinical response to steroids within a week or so, i.e. the patient is feeling significantly better. As we've discussed earlier, PMR symptoms typically resolve quickly. Some GCA symptoms like GCA headache and scalp tenderness also usually improve within a few days. Other GCA symptoms like jaw claudication can take a bit longer and may not resolve for a week or two. Then, over the next few weeks, blood tests should be taken to check that ESR and CRP rates are approaching normal. It's worth mentioning here that, if the PMR patient starts to show signs of having GCA during this period, the steroid dose will be raised and the referral process to the hospital specialist should kick in.

Here we should also mention another aspect of PMR and GCA treatment. Doctors are concerned about the total dose taken over time – we can call this the *cumulative dose*. This is because steroids have long-term as well as short-term risks. A person with PMR starting out on 15mg a day will, by the end of their acute four-week phase, have taken 420mg mg of prednisolone altogether, before starting a taper. A GCA patient starting off on 60mg a day will have taken 1,680mg before starting the taper, i.e. four times as much as the PMR patient. It follows that tapering is a little different depending on whether you have PMR or GCA, and later we give more detailed attention to this.

Ideally, our GPs and rheumatologists would like to see us reduce our daily pred dosage down to zero within a couple of years. There is a growing recognition, however, that this is an unrealistic target for more than half of patients, some of whom will be on steroids for several years. A minority will find that they have to keep taking a small daily dose of prednisolone for the rest of their lives. It's a challenge to unravel the mystery of who these patients are going to turn out to be.

At the beginning of your GCA and PMR journey it's impossible to say whether or not this will be you. Your whole experience of having GCA or PMR may be dogged by uncertainty. We'll come back to the question of tapering with more detail later in the chapter. If we talk first about the many possible side effects and risks of long-term glucocorticoid medication, it will give you a good understanding of why doctors are so keen to get you off them.

Steroid Side effects and consequences

The side effects are legion, both in the short term and as a consequence of being on steroids for a long time. In this section we start with the temporary ones and move on to those that can also have an impact on health going into the future, after you have recovered from PMR or GCA. Psychological disturbances, weight gain, Cushing's syndrome and effects on the eyes may have an impact on your quality of life in the short and medium term. Osteoporosis, glaucoma and cataracts, type II diabetes, and possible depression on withdrawal from the steroids have to be looked out for. The effects on the eyes (glaucoma and cataracts), diabetes, the risk of bone fractures (think increased risk of bone fragility/osteoporosis, plus muscle weakness making you more likely to fall), are likely to be the longer-term side effects that worry doctors most where older people are concerned. Some patients have heard that steroids also affect your risk of developing cardiovascular disease, and we look at the evidence for that. It is important though, to remember that chronic inflammatory illness, if left untreated, can also have a destructive impact on long-term health outcomes.

As if all this were not enough, a whole series of side effects are characterised by medics as being minor. These include nervousness, acne, rashes, increased appetite, hyperactivity, frequent urination, diarrhoea, cramps, and sensitive teeth.

Psychological

Possible early side effects include insomnia, euphoria and, rarely, mania (in particular, in those suffering from bipolar disorders). Pred can also cause symptoms of depression and anxiety in some individuals.

I started off with the euphoria. That was great, and it coincided with Christmas. I felt so happy to be pain-free and able to run around, fully involved with family celebrations. A month later, I had a full-blown breakdown and ended up in bed with my grandson's teddy. It wasn't until years later that a chance remark from Prof. Dasgupta made me think – was that breakdown steroid-induced? I could have been taking more pred than was good for me. I weighed only eight stone and was on a dose that was probably enough for someone half as big again.

Sometimes people can get severe psychological disturbance where they lose contact with reality and may experience delusions or hallucinations termed *steroid-induced psychosis.* Thankfully, proper steroid psychosis is very unusual and generally occurs only at higher doses mainly used for GCA, but other emotional effects of steroids are much more common.

Do talk with your loved ones about the possible effects on your emotions and tell them that, at times, you may have mood swings. You may feel weepy, or perhaps particularly irritable. Insomnia can be a problem. A sensation of 'brain fog' is common. Hmm… where was I? Many of our members in PMRGCAuk and the local support groups have complained about their "steroid head". As a university teacher and manager of a large department, I found this particularly hard, and I am sure brain fog affected my career.

You may have difficulty making decisions. Unfortunately, as many of us are getting on, we might start to think that our lapses of memory and drying up in the middle of a sentence, having completely forgotten what we were going to say, are part of creeping decrepitude. Not so. This is the effect of steroids. Don't give yourself a bad time about it. Just get into the habit of writing things down! Now where did I put that pen?

If we add to this that you may be fed up because you are in pain and worn out because you have not slept very well, we have a pretty explosive mixture. You're fighting a dragon. It's exhausting. You're doing fine. Do not beat yourself up about it if you find you can't be stoical and heroic all the time. Accept yourself.

Do take some time off work to adapt to your diagnosis and your medication. If you are not working, make sure you rest enough. Take special care of yourself. These unpleasant effects may wear off fairly quickly as your body gets used to the drug and the steroid dose reduces. Of course, if they do not wear off, seek help from your GP.

Weight gain and 'moon face'

You may worry about how your appearance may change when you go on steroids. It is bad enough not feeling yourself, so not looking like yourself is adding insult to injury. For some patients this causes huge misery, because it is hard to get used to looking different from your real self as well as feeling like hell. We get this deposit of fat in unwelcome places, like round our middles (our "roid rolls"), the "buffalo hump", or "rhino hump" and the moon face (Cushing's syndrome), while we lose fat and muscle from our upper arms. If PMR or GCA strike during or soon after the menopause, all this change of appearance can be just too much for folks who are barely getting used to the idea of getting older. It is bad enough to have an illness that is supposed to be an illness of the elderly, without changing shape almost overnight.

Dorothy Byrne, former head of news at Channel 4, wrote an article in the Daily Mail about how difficult she found dealing with her changed appearance. As a senior creative in the media industry, she was surrounded by people for whom appearance mattered a lot. Dorothy shared how she found out what doctors think about the side effects of prednisolone:

> *"Doctors call our chubby chops 'moon face'. It's caused partly by water retention, but also by the peculiar way in which steroids redistribute fat round the body. Steroids make takers look puffier because they cause water retention and redistribute fat to the face, back and midriff.*
>
> *"We also have little humps on our backs just below the neck, known as 'buffalo hump'. There is another weird fat deposit round our midriff. Meanwhile, our arms and legs lose muscle and fat. Some medics refer to us as 'lemons on matchsticks'. Others call us 'potatoes on sticks'. Obviously, they don't say these names to our puffy faces."*

A lot of doctors don't mention the likelihood that you'll put on weight. In fact, someone on long-term steroids for PMR or GCA might expect to put on half a stone or more. Doctors tend not to worry so much about moon face and moderate weight gain, and you may get the impression that the doctor thinks you are making a fuss about it. Here, getting in touch with other people, for example through a local support group, or on the web forum, can be tremendously helpful. In the company of your fellow-sufferers you can talk, rant, and laugh about your side effects, knowing you are not alone.

In my own case, I put on a stone (14lb) but it did not bother me too much at the time. My husband was very sweet and reassuring, remarking on my blooming complexion instead of drawing attention to my blooming belly. But once I got better and began to look more like myself before PMR, I could tell by some of the things he said that he was relieved to have me back to my normal self.

Effects on the eyes

You may experience changes in your eyesight while taking steroids, and this can be one of the more worrying side effects. People with PMR may wonder whether GCA is rearing its ugly head, and those with GCA fear a flare and permanent damage to the eye. Certainly, if you get new visual symptoms, especially if they are sudden, severe or getting progressively worse, particularly in one eye, get that checked immediately. However, one common and usually temporary cause of blurring is high blood sugar which can draw extra water into the lens of the eye, slightly altering its shape and changing how it bends light, which causes temporary blurred vision.

If you experience this, you could try cutting down your sugar and refined carbohydrate intake for a day or two and see whether a reduction in your blood sugar has any effect. If it happens frequently, you may need a blood test for diabetes.

Another problem, especially for older people, is glaucoma. Have a regular optician check-up to watch out for this, and for cataracts. Try to get one within six weeks of starting steroids.

Loss of bone density

It has long been known that long-term use of glucocorticoid drugs can lead to a loss of bone density, leading to heightened risk of significant bone thinning (osteoporosis) and fractures. Muscle strength is also affected, adding to risk of falls and fracture. On top of that, inflammatory disease itself has a similar effect. Given that older people are already at a higher risk of fracture than their younger selves, this is pretty important in GCA and PMR patients.

You are between a rock and a hard place, though hopefully, not falling over. You must have enough calcium and vitamin D on board to help counteract these effects. Calcium is one of the main components of bone. Vitamin D helps the body absorb calcium and also helps maintain muscle function and strength, so you are less likely to fall and have that fracture. Prednisolone reduces the amount of calcium you can absorb in your gut, and makes you lose more calcium in your urine, so a supplement is in order. Your doctor may have prescribed a calcium and/or vitamin D3 supplement, such as Adcal or TheiCal. If you tend to eat a lot of calcium rich foods, you may only need to take vitamin D. In sunnier climates, you may get enough vitamin D from sunshine alone, although even here clothing and sun avoidance can limit how much vitamin D the body produces.

Your doctor is also likely to offer you a weekly bisphosphonate medication such as alendronic acid to strengthen your bones. Some are nervous and unwilling to take it, but Vanessa explains below why it's so important and why you might not need to worry too much. If your illness has also led you to take less exercise, particularly walking and other load-bearing exercise which is also important for bone health, you seriously need to consider how to protect your bones. Loss of bone density may be a reason for doctors to prescribe steroid-sparing drugs such as methotrexate.

Vanessa says: on the rationale for taking alendronic acid, or other bisphosphonates

Your bones are constantly renewed by a balance between cells that build bone and cells that break it down. Steroids disrupt this balance by slowing bone formation and increasing bone breakdown, leading to reduced bone density and a much higher risk of osteoporosis and fractures, particularly of the spine (vertebrae) and hips. This risk is especially high in PMR and GCA because treatment usually involves higher doses of steroids for longer periods. Large studies show fracture risk increases by 60–230%, depending on dose and duration, with the greatest risk at doses above 7.5mg daily.

Bisphosphonates have a good safety record and are tolerated by most people. The most common side effects are indigestion, stomach discomfort, or muscle and bone aches. If side effects occur, alternative preparations are available.

They are not the easiest treatments because they must be taken correctly (on an empty stomach with water and staying upright for 30 minutes) and with vitamin D and also calcium if dietary intake is insufficient. But hip and spinal fractures can be life-changing, often leading to long-term pain, reduced mobility, loss of independence and lower quality of life. And I see this in my practice, as rheumatologists are doctors that look after bone health. For this reason, I prescribe a bisphosphonate such as alendronic acid to my PMR and GCA patients for as long as they remain on steroids, unless there is a specific reason not to. These drugs slow bone breakdown and reduce the risk of fractures by about half.

There are two rare side effects of bisphosphonates that people worry about. Osteonecrosis of the jaw (ONJ) is mainly a risk with high-dose intravenous treatment in cancer patients. However, there is probably no greater risk of ONJ in people taking oral bisphosphonates for osteoporosis than those of the same age who don't. The second, atypical fracture of the femur, only occurs in about 2 in 1000 people on treatment for eight to ten years. For most people with PMR and GCA, the benefits of preventing fractures greatly outweigh these very small risks.

---- x ----

Raised blood sugar and diabetes

Steroids play havoc with your body's blood sugar levels. If you were a diabetic before developing PMR or GCA, you do need to be very careful indeed about monitoring your blood sugar levels and keeping them under control by religiously taking your diabetes medication. There is also a lot you can do to help yourself and protect your level of health into the future, by being even stricter about your diet. Try to restrict your refined carbohydrate (sugars) intake as much as you can. If you are relatively young when you get PMR or GCA, a couple of years of relative self-denial will pay dividends in future years by helping to keep your weight and your diabetes under control.

Even if you're not diabetic, you need to be aware of the risks. Diabetes induced by long-term steroid use is a real risk. In a recent survey of patient-reported adverse events in 90 GCA patients in France, one in ten of them reported new diabetes[30].

Normally, insulin tells the liver to reduce how much glucose it releases into the bloodstream and helps muscles and fat take up glucose for energy. Steroids interfere with this process by making the liver, muscles and fat tissues less sensitive to insulin. It doesn't help that the reduced physical activity and weight gain we may experience can make this effect stronger. As a result, the liver continues to release glucose while the body's cells take up less of it. The pancreas responds by producing more and more insulin to try to keep blood sugar under control. Over time, this strain on the system can cause persistently high blood glucose levels and, in some people, this spills over into steroid induced diabetes.

A team at the University of Leeds has for several years been studying the way that being on steroids long-term might affect the health risks of patients with immune-mediated inflammatory diseases (including GCA and PMR). They have been looking at 'big data' drawn from the UK Clinical Practice Research Datalink. This allows researchers to track prescriptions, calculate doses over time, and measure these against medical events, such as new diagnoses and hospital admissions, etc. One study into the risk of Type 2 diabetes for people with no previous history of diabetes took data from 32,593 people with GCA and/or PMR between 1998 and 2017. Imagine a football stadium filled with PMR and GCA patients and you get some idea of the size of this study. It emerged that 8% of the whole research population (over 100,000 patients with various chronic inflammatory diseases treated with steroids) developed diabetes within a follow up period of median five years[31].

What can we do to avoid this happening to us? Well, we need to keep our steroid intake as low as we safely can. We can protect our systems by moderating our diet. Cutting down on foods that cause rapid rises in blood sugar, such as sugary foods and highly refined starchy foods - think white bread, white rice, white pasta, chips, crisps, pastries, pizza bases - can help protect our bodies.

It's a challenge. Often, steroids make us hungrier than we would normally be, and we crave the very things we should eat less of like pastries and chip butties. There's also the temptation to console our poorly selves with treats and calorific comfort eating. I've been there. It's not easy. Plus, if you take in more food than you use, your body stores the extra. Extra weight is also a risk for diabetes, so exercise is another important part of this equation. More about this in Chapter Six.

The researchers concluded that doctors need to make sure that patients are educated about the risk and supported to make changes to their diets, as well as being told about the symptoms of hyperglycaemia (high blood sugar). These include increased thirst, frequent urination, blurred vision, fatigue and weight loss.

As always, I'm not passing this information on to alarm you unduly. If you're like me, you'll tend to think, "Oh, it won't happen to me". But it is going to happen to someone, and that someone *might* be me, or it might be you. Against all my personal expectations (build, fitness, diet, weight, BMI, blood pressure, complacency, etc.) I turned out to have diabetes. Probably I would have got it anyway in the end, but I think I succumbed sooner than I would have done without four and a half years on pred.

I think that my diabetes developed while I was still on steroids, but we didn't realise because I seemed to be getting better (from PMR) and my GP wasn't too worried about me because I wasn't overweight, was active, etc. My "prediabetes" phase was completely missed. It was only when I became quite ill that the diabetes surfaced and he was pretty shocked. He signed me off work for six weeks, which was longer than when I had had the breakdown! So, ask your GP to check you intermittently for a simple blood test called HbA1c that shows your average blood sugar level over the past 2–3 months and picks up pre-diabetes and diabetes.

Gastritis and stomach ulcers

Steroids can make the stomach lining more vulnerable by reducing its natural protective mechanisms. Proton pump inhibitors (PPIs) such as omeprazole or lansoprazole help by reducing stomach acid, which lowers irritation and allows the lining to recover. A PPI is usually prescribed with prednisolone for PMR or GCA from the outset which your doctor might call "stomach protection." Once you get down to less than 10mg daily you can probably stop it unless you have other risk factors for gastric irritation. If you have been on the PPI a while, you may get some rebound indigestion, but that usually settles within a week or two, plus reducing the PPI dose before stopping might help too. If not, you may need to go back on it.

Infection risk

We have a two- to three-fold increased risk of infection, which rises with steroid dose, so it's highest early on in steroid treatment. Most infections are mild, but serious infections can occur, particularly as we get older. Keeping vaccinations up to date, particularly for flu, pneumonia, COVID and shingles, is one of the most effective ways to reduce infection risk while on steroids. Alongside this, it is sensible to take simple measures such as good hand hygiene and avoiding close contact with people who are unwell.

Risk of cardiovascular disease

While it has long been recognised that high doses of steroids over a long period can increase a person's overall risk of heart disease or other cardiovascular conditions, such as aneurysm or stroke, it was also thought that doses of 5mg or less over the long term were relatively safe. However, there was little reliable longitudinal research that followed people up over time. A team at the University of Leeds, in a study looking at whether low to moderate steroid dose increases the risk of cardiovascular disease (CVD), included data from over 25,000 patients with either PMR or GCA or both, who had no prior history of CVD. Their medical records were followed up for a median period of five years.

They found that risk levels for these patients increased dependent on the dosage of steroids they had been taking, even when the inflammatory nature of the illness (disease activity) was taken into account. The risk doubled for people on less than 5mg daily and was no less than six times higher for people whilst on 25mg or more daily[32]. However, there is also evidence that active GCA and, to a lesser extent, PMR may increase cardiovascular risk through chronic inflammation, particularly early on in the illness, so the key aim is tight disease control using the lowest effective steroid dose - the Goldilocks amount. Given that, as we age, increased risk of heart disease is almost inevitable, this is worth being aware of.

Hypertension (high blood pressure) and high cholesterol

High blood pressure is of course a major contributor to heart disease. In another University of Leeds study, this time looking into raised blood pressure over time, it turned out that both the daily dose and the cumulative dosage of steroids increased risk[33].

Cholesterol changes are a current daily dose effect, not a cumulative-dose effect. That said, having high cholesterol increases long term cardiovascular risk, as does high blood pressure and diabetes, even if they go away after we stop steroids. It's a case of damage done that may come back to hit us later – a true sting in the tail of the dragon.

Side effects and tapering your steroid dose

Let's just recap here. If doctors follow the guidelines, then tapering for PMR and GCA will start from a wide range of doses from 12.5 to 60mg, so the shape and length of the taper will differ depending on that starting dose, even if the person doesn't relapse along the way. The resulting risk of steroid side effects will differ in line with this. We know from research that the rate of steroid side effects is closely linked to the daily dose and also the cumulative dose of steroid that the person has had.

Some things like mood and sleep disturbance and sugar levels in the body are most affected by the daily dose, whilst other side effects like bone fragility and cataracts are a result of the cumulative dose. The more steroid side effects a person actually develops, the keener the doctor will be to push down the steroid dose (speed up the taper) to minimise those side effects, i.e. sailing closer to the wind. Of course, sailing closer to the wind means that person is more likely to flare. And getting the balance right between these two things can be tricky, especially if the person doesn't have easy access to the doctor again, or clear advice about what to do if flare does happen.

Glucocorticoid Induced Adrenal Insufficiency (GIAI)

Prednisolone is chemically related to the hormone cortisol, a glucocorticoid which the normal healthy body manufactures in the adrenal gland. It is a vital hormone that helps the body respond to stress, regulate inflammation, maintain normal blood pressure and blood sugar levels, and support normal day-to-day functioning. Cortisol production mainly happens during the hours of daylight, with a peak first thing in the morning and much lower levels during the night. Taking prednisolone suppresses this natural process so that the adrenal gland does not produce as much of the body's natural cortisol as before and may reduce production really significantly. Thus, it may be dangerous if steroids are withdrawn too quickly or stopped suddenly. This is termed glucocorticoid-induced adrenal insufficiency (GI-AI, or adrenal suppression for short).

Endocrinologists (that's hormone specialists to you and me) say that adrenal suppression can occur if prednisolone is taken for longer than 3-4 weeks. As long as patients continue to take their prescribed steroid, this is usually not harmful (although read on to find the section on what to do if you become really unwell). Problems arise if the dose is reduced too quickly for the body to recover its natural cortisol production, especially around 5mg daily, which is similar to normal body levels of cortisol. The prednisolone dose has come down below the body's usual requirements, but the adrenal gland has not yet recovered enough to take up the slack.

Low levels of natural cortisol, without enough prednisolone on board to counteract the shortage, can cause many symptoms, including chronic fatigue and weakness, muscular pains, weight loss, stomach upset, vomiting, headache and low blood pressure.

This is why the dosage should be gradually reduced, to give the body time to restart its own cortisol production, while also keeping the PMR or GCA safely under control. This weaning process may be over a few days, if the course of prednisolone was short, but may take weeks or months if the patient has been on long-term treatment, as in PMR and GCA.

In a large study from Norwich in the UK[34], which looked at several hundred people with GCA, only 4% (roughly 1 in 25) of patients went on to develop adrenal insufficiency that was significant enough to require long term steroid replacement. That is an important figure: it tells us that persistent, clinically meaningful adrenal "failure" does occur, but only in a small minority.

In a large Danish study of people with PMR and GCA, patients were assessed after they had stopped prednisolone[35]. Only 1.9% (about 1 in 50) had confirmed adrenal insufficiency on formal testing. But at the same time, 34% (around 1 in 3) reported symptoms that are typically associated with adrenal insufficiency such as fatigue, weakness, and poor physical function.

So, if only around 1-4% of patients have true long term adrenal insufficiency, why do so many more, as many as 1 in 3 of us, *feel* as though we do?

The Danish study itself provides a possible key to resolving this. It showed that people with symptoms often had slightly lower cortisol levels, even if they did not meet the formal threshold for adrenal insufficiency. In other words, their bodies were not fully back to normal, but they were also not in true adrenal insufficiency. Alongside this, symptoms were linked to reduced muscle strength, higher body fat, and poorer physical performance, suggesting that perhaps the effects of long-term steroid use on the body, including deconditioning and muscle loss, play a role too.

Your adrenal glands aren't so much an on-off switch as an "on-demand" system where there might be a bit of a lag between the demands of your life and the adrenal response. This is just a way of saying that these last months coming off steroids may have some good days and some not-so-good days, and it's part of the process of your body adjusting.

Adrenal crisis

Patients are justifiably concerned about an "adrenal crisis" occurring if someone has GIAI and cannot take prednisolone for some reason, or due to an acute stress when the body cannot produce enough additional cortisol to meet increased demands. It is a potentially life-threatening medical emergency that must be treated immediately with steroid medication and occurs when the body cannot produce enough cortisol to deal with a stress situation. Some patients with confirmed adrenal insufficiency carry an emergency injection of hydrocortisone in case of a crisis happening and wear a steroid alert bracelet.

When should you think about this? If you are on a lower dose (around 10mg or less), you may need to increase it during significant illness (often roughly doubling), whereas at higher doses (around 15–20mg or more) you usually already have enough steroid, but should still seek advice if you are very unwell. You may also be given specific advice about increasing your dose for operations, and if you are unable to keep tablets down you may need urgent treatment with injectable steroids. Doctors define "significant illness" as things like a high fever or infection needing antibiotics, not a cold or feeling a bit under the weather. This advice is sometimes called "sick day rules."

Steroid withdrawal syndrome (SWS)

Regardless of what steroid dose you are on, it's also not that uncommon to get withdrawal symptoms for a few days after the dose is dropped. This isn't happening because the body is short of cortisol, but because it has adapted to having the higher dose of steroid on board and needs time to adjust. Think of it like stepping from bright sunlight into a darker room; your eyes don't adjust immediately. At first, everything seems dim, even though the light levels are fine. Symptoms of steroid withdrawal include feeling tired, achy, low in mood, or generally unwell, and people sometimes also notice symptoms such as headaches, dizziness, nausea, poor appetite, disturbed sleep, or a general sense of weakness.

Adrenal insufficiency and steroid withdrawal share similar symptoms, but they are thought to be different things that often overlap until the body's natural hormone regulation finally recovers after coming off steroids. To complicate things further, you may also have noticed that many of their symptoms are quite similar to those of PMR and GCA!

Paying attention to timing may help differentiate steroid withdrawal (and adrenal insufficiency) from flare: symptoms tend to come on soon after a dose drop, then lift over a few days. But the most honest bottom line is that in real life these three things can be hard to distinguish at steroid doses of less than say 5-7.5mg daily.

Prednisolone also lowers the body's production of another adrenal hormone called DHEA (*Dehydroepiandrosterone*). Because DHEA plays a role in energy levels, mood, concentration and sex drive, this might possibly help to explain why some people on long-term prednisolone feel unusually tired, flat in mood, or notice a reduced libido (remember libido?), even when their inflammatory disease is well controlled. However, this is probably only part of the picture, and not a complete explanation for steroid withdrawal symptoms or adrenal insufficiency.

This knowledge is quite new, and more research is needed for doctors to understand these processes better.

So, to recap, feeling unwell during steroid tapering is common and real, but in most cases, it reflects a broader recovery process caused by years on the drug rather than permanently reduced adrenal function. A small minority develop true adrenal insufficiency and need ongoing replacement, while a much larger group, perhaps up to a third of us, experience symptoms that may be due to a combination of steroid withdrawal syndrome, gradual adrenal recovery, physical deconditioning, and the underlying disease. Every attempt to reduce below a lowish threshold brings on a rush of pain, malaise and discomfort. The intuitive response is to go back up to the dose at which you were comfortable. But then you never manage to come off the pred, keeping yourself on a lowish dose for years.

Many people in online groups report they have adrenal insufficiency following years on pred and need to take a maintenance dose of a few milligrams per day to compensate for the cortisol that their body isn't making naturally. If you find yourself wondering whether this is you, do give yourself a chance to reduce the steroids to zero or near-zero. It might be worth a few weeks' relative discomfort if you find you actually can come off altogether. Why not try a "smooth and slow" taper to help you do it? More on this in the next chapter.

You can also ask your GP or rheumatologist whether a morning cortisol test might be helpful. Doctors advise that this should be done 24 hours after your last dose, i.e. about 9 am, before your daily dose of pred, at about 4mg pred or less. If you have the test on a higher dose, in most people on long term steroids, it will be low.

Remember, that's OK because you are taking enough prednisolone to compensate. The test is only helpful when you get to steroid doses lower than about 4mg daily.

The European Society for Endocrinology (ESE) has recently published a patient education leaflet on glucocorticoid-induced adrenal insufficiency, based on their new international guideline for clinicians. They say, "For most people, gradually tapering off glucocorticoids will result in normalisation of your body's ability to produce cortisol"[36]. I welcome the publication of the ESE clinical guideline, because it is helpful for rheumatologists and shows medicine working across specialisms. It also reflects my own experience. Coming off steroids was really difficult, but I kept telling myself that if I was going to live at least another thirty years, I blooming well had to do it.

Perhaps if there was more attention given by doctors to these closing stages of the fight with the dragon, and more understanding of the sting in the tail, it would be possible to support more patients to work through the stage of steroid withdrawal syndrome/adrenal suppression to a final point of coming off the prednisolone completely.

It also suggests that those people who find that they really can't get off the steroids and are stuck with taking, say, 5mg a day indefinitely, are simply replacing the physiological cortisol that they are not making any more now that their adrenals have packed up.

Summing up

We have taken a good look at the side effects of pred, both more or less immediate, and long-term. It's a fair bet that almost everyone on steroids for GCA or PMR will experience some of them. For most of us it's a trade-off between relief from the symptoms of disease and the discomfort of side effects. However, we also need to be mindful of the effects of a high cumulative dose after years on steroids, affecting all parts of our body, including our vital organs and systems.

Adrenal insufficiency is a sting in the tail of PMR or GCA that we need to be aware of. However, it's important not to assume that symptoms are always due to adrenal insufficiency alone because steroid withdrawal symptoms can overlap with it. In practice, these experiences can be difficult to disentangle. With a slow taper, both usually can be got through, although some discomfort along the way is not uncommon.

It's not just a question of moderating as much as possible the daily doses that patients are taking but also reducing as much as possible the length of time that people are on steroids. This of course can be really difficult, especially when your condition refuses to play ball, and it is well known that some unlucky people end up on a low dose of steroids pretty much permanently.

Doctors have to take the 'big data' into account when making judgments about the degree of risk of prescribing for you. They also need to consider any 'co-morbidities' you have, i.e. those other long-term conditions that are almost expected as we age, like blood pressure that gradually creeps upwards by itself. You also need to think about the degree of risk you personally feel comfortable with.

This new understanding of the cumulative impact of long-term steroid medication is also really important for arguing the case for alternatives to prednisolone for treating PMR and GCA, at *all* levels of severity. We can now move on to the nitty-gritty of how you reduce your steroid dose down to the lowest possible level for you.

4: Tapering steroids

Everyone is expected to taper their dose of steroids, reducing gradually to zero or near zero. By the end of this chapter, I hope you'll be clear that, if you don't fit the simplified version of the journey through steroid treatment, you're not abnormal in any way. You share this with at least half of other patients.

After being on steroid medication for more than a few weeks, your body becomes reliant on the drug because its own natural steroid production is suppressed. For this reason, you should never stop taking prednisolone suddenly once you have been on treatment for more than 3-4 weeks. The dose must always be tapered or reduced gradually over time to control the disease while allowing the body's natural cortisol production to recover and minimise side effects.

When tapering, you have to be aware of several things that might be happening at once. First, how well your symptoms are being controlled by the dose you are on; next, what side effects you're experiencing. Then, what happens when you try to reduce your dose. You may be able to reduce easily and smoothly, as on the schedule from the doctor. You may experience flaring. Flares are a major concern both for patients and doctors, and so we're going to talk about them before we get into the nuts and bolts of tapering. If you are lucky, you may avoid flares altogether, but it's well-nigh impossible to reliably predict who will flare and who won't.

As you reduce, you may also experience withdrawal symptoms, and/or adrenal insufficiency. We will look more closely at each of these later in the chapter. It can be difficult to tell what is happening and when, because the signs and symptoms of all of these can be quite similar. It's easy to think that you need to raise your dose to where it was when you last felt symptom-free. But read on. Even this may not be as straightforward as it seems.

Flares

As we have noted, a flare is a return of disease activity to a level where you feel it, i.e. no longer controlled by the medication. A PMR flare is usually a return of the same kind of symptoms felt at the start of the illness, that inflammatory pain and stiffness in the shoulder and hip girdles, but it does not have to be identical in pattern or severity to the first episode.

GCA flare means a return of GCA symptoms but again, not necessarily following the same pattern as at first diagnosis. Symptoms may be similar to last time, but hopefully milder because the person now recognises them and can act on them immediately. The most common symptoms at GCA flare are headache, the emergence of PMR symptoms, and “constitutional upset”, which is an umbrella term doctors use to describe general signs of being unwell, such as weight loss and night sweats. An interesting study found that in GCA, isolated PMR features were much more common at relapse (46%) than at initial diagnosis (10%), while isolated headache was less common at relapse (20% vs 66% at diagnosis). High inflammatory blood markers are also a typical feature. In fact, a flare could be signalled by a significant increase in your inflammatory markers in a blood test, with no other obvious cause.

This raises the question whether bloods should be monitored regularly throughout the taper. If you are feeling well, one could argue that regular blood tests aren't needed because ‘how’ you are feeling is most important. However, monitoring CRP and/or ESR adds extra information. CRP and/or ESR are usually (but not always) up during relapses. It's often useful for the doctor to look at the pattern of the CRP or ESR over time. Has the initial high level been nice and suppressed for some time until the last few readings where it has been rising sequentially, in line with you feeling less well? Certain other aspects of your blood count can also help. For example, people can become anaemic when their PMR or GCA is not under control. Normal inflammatory markers make a flare less likely and alert the doctor to consider other cause(s) for your symptoms. It's important to note that raised CRP and ESR are not specific to PMR and GCA, and can go up with any kind of inflammation, for example an infection.

If you flare, don't feel that somehow you are getting it wrong - unfortunately for many it's a typical part of the disease process. This rather gives the impression that, while steroids are very effective at controlling symptoms most of the time, the balancing act of maintaining the Goldilocks amount while steadily tapering, is a Holy Grail.

Vanessa says: on tapering and flare

I use the BSR steroid reduction regimens for PMR and GCA as a starting point but explain right at the beginning that most people need to adapt the taper as they go along and that's expected and that's okay, as no one size fits all. Someone who comes down the taper without any adjustments is one of the lucky ones in my practice, although as a rheumatologist I only see the GCA patients and the difficult-to-treat PMR patients, so may have a skewed view.

If someone has a flare or is struggling, then the basic principles of steroid adjustment are often the same for PMR and for GCA. A reasonable Plan A for flare management is to increase to 5mg above the last level that controlled symptoms for a week, then drop to the last level that controlled symptoms (not the level of flare), then consider whether tapering a bit more slowly might be helpful.

If a person with PMR subsequently develops GCA, they will need to start the GCA taper from the beginning (40-60mg daily).

In those with GCA, if clear "ischaemic" symptoms occur at flare such as convincing GCA visual symptoms or transient ischaemic attack (TIA or transient stroke symptoms), then it will often be necessary to go back up to a high starting dose again to protect from permanent sight loss or stroke. Thankfully that's not that common. But even that may be individualised. Imagine a GCA patient who flares with symptoms including jaw pain on chewing (i.e., jaw claudication, considered an ischaemic symptom of GCA), but their bloods do not show much inflammation and the ultrasound of their temporal and axillary arteries is normal (when the bloods and ultrasound had been very abnormal at the outset). Plus, this person was very anxious and couldn't sleep on higher doses of prednisolone and now has diabetes and hypertension. Then we may agree for them to first try 10mg higher than the level that previously controlled symptoms, with a clear plan to seek urgent medical advice if they don't quickly improve over 24-48 hours. I would also discuss starting a steroid-sparing medication or "DMARD" (Disease Modifying Antirheumatic Drug) to lower the risk of future flares and reduce the future steroid burden.

However, the plan for this patient comes with a disclaimer because guidelines suggest going back to 60mg as jaw claudication is a GCA symptom associated with sight loss. But guidelines are blunt tools that cannot provide an individualised approach based on the whole clinical picture and don't take into consideration the person's attitude to risk.

---- x ----

Factors your doctor might be considering at flare

When your doctor advises on how to manage a flare and adjust your steroid taper, Vanessa says they are quietly weighing up many factors, including:

- How active your disease is at the moment. In GCA, this is classed as major or minor relapse; in PMR, it is less clearly defined, usually supported by raised inflammatory markers on blood tests.
- The dose of steroid you are on now.
- Your overall disease history, including how many flares you have had, how long you have been ill, your total lifetime steroid exposure, and whether you have had large-vessel or ischaemic GCA.
- Other illnesses that can mimic PMR or GCA symptoms. How confident are they that you are actually having a flare?
- How badly steroids have affected you so far, both the severity and the number of side effects.
- Other medical conditions affected by steroids, such as diabetes, high blood pressure or mental health problems.
- Symptoms from steroid withdrawal.
- Evidence of steroid-induced adrenal suppression.
- Other stresses in your life, such as illness, bereavement or emotional strain.
- Your own and your doctor's attitude to risk and fear of flare.
- Access to tocilizumab in GCA. In the cases where Vanessa knows she will be able to obtain NHS funding for tocilizumab, she tapers the steroid more steeply than she used to, in the knowledge she can reach for tocilizumab if needed. Once on tocilizumab she can then taper more quickly, often twice as fast, which is one of the main reasons she uses it.
- Whether you are on other immune-suppressing drugs (DMARDs), which may reduce flare risk even if they do not always allow faster tapering.
- Your body weight.
- Your ability to manage a more complex taper, such as alternate-day dosing.

All this is very complicated to get your head around. It might be an interesting exercise and actually really useful in practice for you to go through this list at home, perhaps with a friend or partner, and think about whether there's anything in particular you'd like to share with the doctor at your next appointment.

So now, having paid due attention to the possibility or even likelihood that your taper may not be as smooth as you and your doctor would like it to be, let's consider what the taper actually looks like, according to the medical guidelines for treating GCA and PMR.

Tapering steroids in GCA

Because GCA needs a much higher starting dose than PMR, at between 40mg and 60mg a day, the initial drops are bigger, to get your dose down to a maintenance level. And the taper takes longer. International guidelines are all quite similar. Here is the GCA taper suggested by the British Society of Rheumatology:

A. Once in clinical remission, reduce the daily dose by 10mg every 2 weeks down to 20mg, then

B. reduce the daily dose by 2.5mg every 2-4 weeks down to 10mg, then

C. reduce the daily dose by 1mg every 1-2 months

If you find you're OK with this reduction, by all means carry on, and get down to 10mg a day as soon as you can do it without flaring.

In the figure below, we see what the reduction might look like if a GCA patient were following the taper as outlined in the guidelines, if (from 20mg) they reduce every 4 weeks. The vertical axis shows the daily dose of prednisolone in mg, and the solid line shows the taper. The dotted line is an imagined representation of the way that the disease activity is also reducing but always controlled by the drug. In other words, the steroids are always on top of the disease activity.

We can see that, despite the drops being large, it takes a full five months to get down to 10mg per day. Dropping every 2 weeks from 20mg would still take three months.

Please note that in the charts that follow, I am illustrating a level of dose with an *imagined* level of disease activity trundling along with the effect of the steroids.

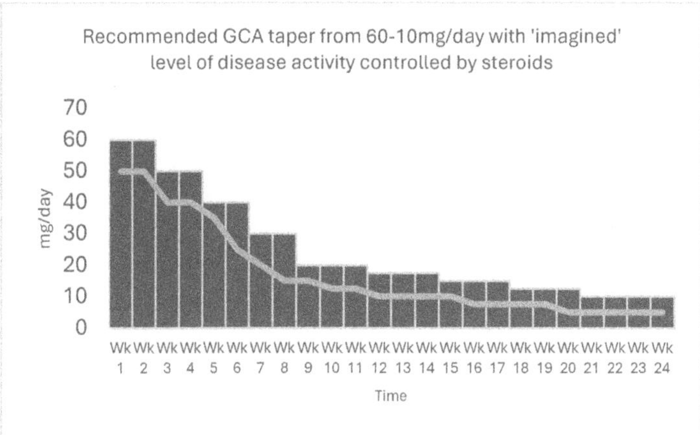

Figure 1: Line chart showing BSR-recommended GCA taper over approx. 6 months to 10 mg with an 'imagined' level of disease activity controlled by the steroids

Medical orthodoxy seems to be that once GCA is under control, it shouldn't be too difficult to reduce the steroid dose in the early days of treatment. The priority is to blitz the inflammation in the arteries with prednisolone and then bring the dose down pretty rapidly. But not everyone finds it easy to drop down to 10mg a day after having been on 40-60mg for weeks. It can be particularly difficult when people who started on high doses have reduced to some extent, but then when they try to drop further, pain and stiffness and just plain unwellness come back. It feels like the dragon has come out and is lurching and pouncing and breathing fire again.

This might be because you have flaring GCA, and of course that's important to discuss with your rheumatologist, but what may be happening is steroid withdrawal. Symptoms of illness return, but they are not the same symptoms as full-blown GCA in the acute early stage. You may feel much more tired, achy and run down. The clue here is that steroid withdrawal symptoms tend to come on immediately after a dose drop and then slowly lift over a few days.

In GCA and also PMR, it might suit you personally to smooth the taper at these high doses (with agreement from your doctor) by taking smaller steps, rather than making a single jump down all in one go. For example, 5mg every week rather than 10mg every fortnight, or 1mg every 1-2 weeks rather than 2.5mg every 2-4 weeks. The rate (speed) of taper is not that affected, but the whole process is gentler and smoother. Be aware, though, that this might increase your cumulative dose slightly.

Vanessa says: on the guidelines for tapering

The 2020 BSR GCA guidelines recommend attempting to taper over 12-18 months providing there is no relapse, defined as return of GCA symptoms, signs or laboratory markers of inflammation[37]*. This tends to be misquoted and misinterpreted as "treatment should be given for 12-18 months" and if that doesn't happen it's somehow "atypical" or "wrong."*

However, studies looking at real-world groups of GCA patients suggest that most GCA patients stay on steroids much longer than recommended, with a mean (average) treatment duration exceeding two years. The mean is the mid-point, so half of people take steroids for less than the mean time point and half take them for longer than the mean time point, i.e. more than half of people with GCA take steroids for MORE than two years. These studies show that steroid treatment is generally required for 1-3 years, with a substantial minority (approximately 25-40% depending on the group of GCA patients studied) needing treatment for over 5 years.

In PMR, the real-world pattern is very similar. The mean time on steroids is 2 years (so half need steroids for MORE than two years) and 25% are on steroids for over 4 years even though guidelines suggest a taper that lasts about a year.

So, there is a disconnect between what is recommended and what actually happens. I've been discussing this with experts Professor Toby Helliwell and Dr Sarah Mackie, and we agree that the reasons for this are probably quite complicated. Published studies of real-world patients suggest that relapse rate in GCA is about 50%. And some people have flary GCA, so will have multiple flares needing adjustment of their taper.

Relapse is very common in PMR too with an estimated rate of about 40% by one year. But this wouldn't explain all the difference. Perhaps it's because people stay on a certain dose for longer because of unreported flare symptoms, steroid withdrawal symptoms, or concerns about the possibility of flaring, or because of other things happening in their lives like infections. Perhaps they simply can't get prompt advice from their GP or rheumatologist about tapering. Some people with PMR and or GCA need steroids for the rest of their lives: some for chronic PMR/GCA and some for long-term steroid-induced adrenal insufficiency.

None of this is the person's fault, although sadly people are often somehow made to feel that it is.

---- x ----

Tapering steroids in PMR

All PMR and GCA management guidelines say every patient should have an individualised plan to taper their dose towards zero. With that caveat, recognising people are different, they suggest a *recommended* tapering regime for PMR would be:

A. Initial tapering: Taper dose to an oral dose of 10 mg/day prednisolone equivalent within 4–8 weeks. So, if the starting dose was 15mg/day, then after 2-4 weeks on that dose, the dose would drop to 12.5mg/day for 2-4 weeks, then drop to 10mg/day.

B. Relapse therapy (if needed): Increase oral prednisolone to the pre-relapse dose and decrease it gradually (within 4–8 weeks) to the dose at which the relapse occurred.

C. Tapering once remission is achieved (following initial and relapse therapies): Taper daily oral prednisolone by 1 mg every 4-8 weeks, (or by 1.25mg reductions using schedules such as 10/7.5 mg alternate days, etc) until discontinuation given that remission is maintained.

This is the European guideline advice, but all the international guidelines are pretty similar.

In the UK, prednisolone is available orally as 5mg, 2.5mg or 1mg tablets, which allows for very fine adjustment of doses. The 1mg dose isn't available in some countries, so doctors and patients there have to be a little creative in 'tailoring' small dose changes, say at 6 or 8mg a day.

For a PMR patient who follows the regime above, dropping by 1mg per month once they get to 10mg/day, and doesn't have any flares, we could envisage a situation like this, in which the prednisolone dosage stays on top of the symptoms of the disease all the way through. This is what your doctor would like to see. A nice steady downward slope.

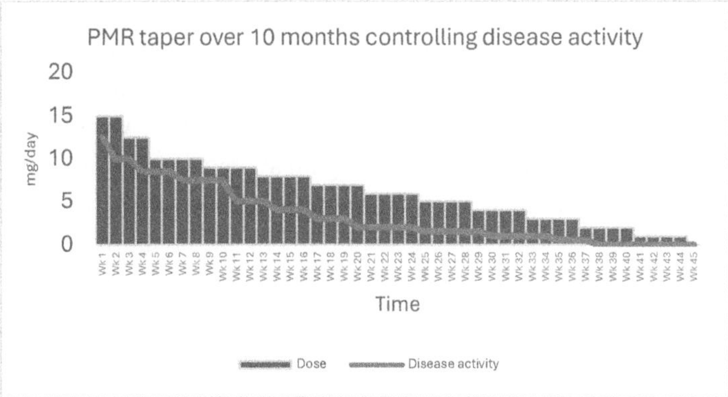

Figure 2: Line chart of 'ideal' PMR taper controlling disease

As you see, this would lead to recovery and stopping the medication within a year. The disease activity is steadily decreasing at the same rate as the drug taper, always under the level that the steroids can control. This is what medics call "clinical remission". All well and good. Except that we can't assume that the underlying condition, the PMR, is playing ball and reducing activity. The glucocorticoids are just dampening down the excess inflammation in the body. If the dosage goes down so low and so quickly that it can't manage the PMR, symptoms will return, a flare. We know that the majority of PMR patients are on steroids for well over a year, so the patients who are able to reduce to zero on this recommended taper are a minority.

If the slower taper is used for PMR or the person has GCA and is on the GCA taper, i.e. coming down from higher, then it will take longer. But we know that most rheumatologists accept that it will take *at least* one to two years for patients to come off steroids, which implies they assume that there will be flary disease for many. The speed of steroid tapering is the main predictor of relapse for PMR and for GCA. One solution would be to give an extra-long taper from the outset to minimise the risk, but then of course steroid side effects could be unacceptable.

Figure 3 is a version that shows how a patient may start to relapse or flare as the dosage is brought down to the point where the disease gets going again, meaning that the year goes by without them being able to reduce much. We see flares around week 9, week 17, a definite spike around week 25, and again at around week 30. This patient is spending a good proportion of the time with the underlying condition not being controlled by the prednisolone. By week 33 there's acceptance that the dosage needs to be kept stable for a while. To be fair, this illustration maybe exaggerates the randomness of flary PMR, but I wanted to show that things can get a bit out of hand.

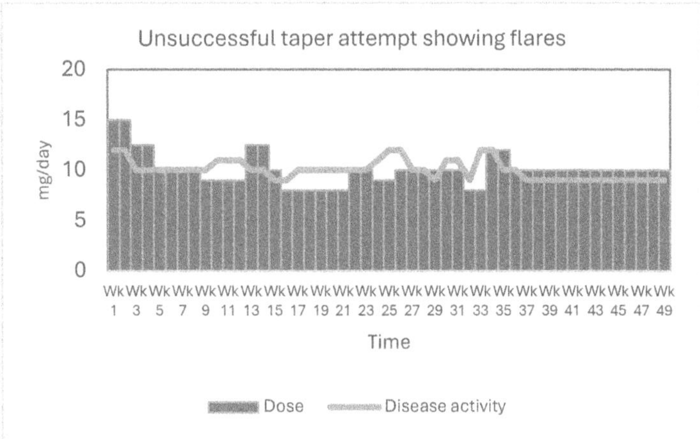

Figure 3: Line chart showing unsuccessful taper with uncontrolled PMR over almost a year

Getting down to lower doses

On on-line forums like HealthUnlocked, people frequently report that small dose reductions feel larger at lower doses. When you think about it, a drop from 8 to 7mg is just about twice as big a drop, proportionately, as one from 15 to 14, so perhaps it's no wonder we have trouble. The further down we go, the bigger a drop of a single milligram gets, as a proportion of what we were taking before. At the first international symposium on PMR and GCA, held in Chelmsford, Essex in 2012, Prof. Wolfgang Schmidt, a German specialist who pioneered the use of ultrasound for GCA diagnosis and the concept of GCA fast track pathways, said he puts his patients on a very gradual reduction indeed. This struck a chord with me and made a lot of sense.

His patients, when getting down from 8mg to 7mg daily, spend a week with six days on 8mg and one on 7mg. The next week, five days on 8mg and two on 7mg (not together, say, Sunday and Tuesday). And so on until the whole week is on 7mg per day. This means that the reduction is a bit slower, but the body gets fooled into not really noticing the drop and adapts itself to the lower dose. This is also an effective way to allow the adrenal glands that have been dormant during steroid treatment to switch back on when the dose gets really low, less than about 5mg per day.

A variant is illustrated in the table below. If you think this kind of reduction programme might suit you, and prevent you from having flares and suffering pain and stiffness while reducing, why not discuss it with your doctor?

Vanessa says: on approaches to tapering below 10mg

There is no one correct way to reduce below 10mg daily, as long as you do it slowly at a rate no faster than 1mg per month. Faster than this and there is a higher risk that your GCA or PMR will flare, plus you will probably feel unwell as you have not given your body or your adrenal glands time to catch up with the reducing prednisolone dose. You may need to go slower, say at 0.5mg per month, especially below about 5 mg daily. Here are a couple of ways to do it. The first is to reduce the dose like coming down a staircase, dropping to the new dose, staying there for a month then dropping to the new lower dose. Table 1 below shows reducing 0.5mg each month.

Some people find that they feel less well the few days after each dose drop, even with 0.5 mg drops. They prefer to use the reduction shown in Table 2, where the ***total weekly dose*** *reduces by 1 mg. This way, the dose comes down at about the same rate, but the reduction is smoother. This is less like a staircase and more like a slope, and some patients report this feels more comfortable because there are no sudden drops.*

Dose	*Tablets needed*
5 mg daily	*5 mg*
4.5 mg daily	*2.5 mg + 1 mg +1mg or* *5mg one day, 4mg the next, alternating*
4 mg daily	*1mg + 1 mg + 1 mg +1 mg*
3.5 mg daily	*2.5 mg + 1 mg or* *4 mg one day, 3 mg the next, alternating*
3 mg daily	*1mg + 1 mg + 1 mg*
2.5 mg daily	*2.5 mg or 3 mg one day, 2 mg the next, alternating*
2 mg daily	*1 mg + 1 mg*
1.5 mg daily	*2 mg one day, 1 mg the next, alternating*
1 mg daily	*1 mg*
0.5 mg daily	*1 mg alternate days. Then STOP*

Table 1: Step wise reduction from 5mg daily, dropping by 0.5 mg per month

Week	Mon	Tue	Wed	Thu	Fri	Sat	Sun	Weekly total	Avg. daily dose
Week 0	5 mg	5 mg	5 mg	5 mg	5 mg	5 mg	5 mg	35 mg	5.00 mg
Week 1	5 mg	5 mg	4 mg	5 mg	5 mg	5 mg	5 mg	34 mg	4.86 mg
Week 2	4 mg	5 mg	4 mg	5 mg	5 mg	5 mg	5 mg	33 mg	4.71 mg
Week 3	4 mg	5 mg	4 mg	5 mg	4 mg	5 mg	5 mg	32 mg	4.57 mg
Week 4	4 mg	5 mg	4 mg	5 mg	4 mg	5 mg	4 mg	31 mg	4.43 mg
Week 5	4 mg	5 mg	4 mg	4 mg	4 mg	5 mg	4 mg	30 mg	4.29 mg
Week 6	4 mg	4 mg	4 mg	4 mg	4 mg	5 mg	4 mg	29 mg	4.14 mg
Week 7	4 mg	4 mg	4 mg	4 mg	4 mg	4 mg	4 mg	28 mg	4.00 mg

Table 2: An example of a smooth slow taper dropping 1mg over 7 weeks (a version of DSNS), then repeat to drop from 4mg to 3mg and so on

This slowed and smoothed-out rather than stepwise taper, or a version of it, has been dubbed the DSNS taper system by PMRPro, patient volunteer on the HealthUnlocked forum. It stands for Dead Slow Nearly Stop. Once down to a few milligrams, some people who have been on steroids several years, may need to go slower, staying at each weekly dose for more than one week.

Smoothing the taper at higher doses won't need these micro reductions. For example, 50 for two weeks dropping to 40 may be too much of a drop for some people with GCA, but going back to 50, then dropping from 50 to 45 then to 40 every 1 to 2 weeks may be fine.

It is important that you discuss your planned steroid taper with your doctor. I tend to give people control over their taper, but with guard rails. While I am usually happy for my patients to control the "smoothness", I do like to help plan the slowness, i.e., the overall rate of dose reduction. The activity of your PMR/GCA, the steroid side effects you have experienced, the time you have been on steroids, the current dose you are taking, your other health problems, and any additional medications you take are just some of the things that may affect how quickly it is safe and sensible to reduce your dose.

---- x ----

There are no good studies establishing the "best" steroid tapering regimen, but you have to start somewhere, so the starting dose and taper schedules outlined in national and international guidelines are a tried and tested reasonable plan A, as long as it's accepted that you may need to adjust the dose at some point along the way.

Unfortunately, it's not usually possible from someone's symptoms at the outset to know when, by how much, or how often they will need to do that, because PMR and GCA (and how the body responds to steroids) can be so different in different people, which is probably why a one-size-fits-all steroid taper has not been developed.

The rheumatology community continues to be very concerned about the burden of long-term steroids on the body. There is a school of thought that a sizeable proportion of PMR patients will not be relapsers and could potentially come off steroids within six months of control of symptoms. This hasn't found its way into widespread practice, but there is a rationale emerging that a shorter taper could be tried. Some people would be symptom-free, and could come off medication. For those who aren't and can't, alternatives to steroids could be made available. The over-arching principle here would be to reduce the overall cumulative load of steroids in all PMR patients as much as possible. But a caveat to this idea is that there is *no* fixed timeframe for PMR and there is no one-size-fits-all taper. We hope this faster taper might benefit those who can reduce steroids more quickly, while prompting earlier rheumatology referral for those who cannot, *without* implying that all PMR patients should stop steroids within six months. Tapering has to be tailored to the individual. Basically, everyone wants the same thing, the Goldilocks amount.

Problems with tapering

Have you been having trouble getting down below 10mg per day of prednisolone? If so, you are not alone! The massive number of posts about tapering on the PMRGCAuk HealthUnlocked internet forum are an eloquent witness of the struggles people have with getting their steroid intake down and keeping it down.

Coming down from the initial higher doses for PMR and even for GCA may not be so difficult, but once we are down below 15mg, things may start to get harder. Many of us discover that when we try reducing from, say, 8mg to 7mg, all our symptoms seem to come back with a vengeance. You might wonder if you are having a flare, or whether this is your body complaining about getting a lower dose. This can be a stage in the journey of PMR and GCA when you may feel particularly alone. This is not what the doctor told you would happen. Up to now, you were doing so well. Now, you have stopped being a "good" patient. You ache, you can't turn over in bed, you feel wiped out. What is going wrong?

It's quite likely you are one of those PMR and/or GCA patients whose experience of tapering doesn't follow the textbook route, and this might be why you are reading this book. Between 10 and 7 mg a day seems to be a sticking point for many. You try the lower dose and symptoms return. You up it again. After a month you try to reduce again. No luck. This is *yo-yo-ing.*

During the taper, almost everyone will experience symptoms at some time or another. These can be a return of former pains, or new pains or just feeling generally unwell. It's always a bit of a riddle whether these symptoms are due to a flare, to steroid withdrawal or steroid-induced adrenal insufficiency. And it might be other health problems rearing their head too, such as the pain and stiffness from osteoarthritis or weaker muscles from months or years on steroids.

Here are some quotes from our PMRGCAuk awareness patient group talking about the uncertainty and confusion around their PMR/GCA journey:

> *"I always feel that there is an imbalance between how my body actually reacts and how it's meant to react."*
>
> *"Is it the taking or the tapering of steroids that's giving me symptoms?"*
>
> *"Is it the disease, the treatment or the tapering that's making me ill?"*
>
> *"I just don't know if steroids are my enemy or my friend, it's all very confusing."*

These words resonate strongly with me. There is still so much uncertainty around PMR and GCA, not only for patients but for doctors too. I would have hoped that things might have improved a good deal over the last fifteen years. And in some ways, they have, but that sense of insecurity and doubt still hangs around.

A general rule of thumb is if you feel awful the day after you reduce your dose and it lifts within a few days, then it's likely that your body has noticed the drop in steroid dose and it is steroid withdrawal or maybe adrenal insufficiency. If it takes a few days or more before you feel unwell, there's a higher chance it's a flare.

One relatively simple way to judge whether you are having a flare or experiencing the discomfort of steroid withdrawal can be to try taking paracetamol (Tylenol in US) for the pain. If it's steroid withdrawal, the painkillers might help. If it's the PMR/GCA dragon rearing its head again, they probably won't.

There are two specific situations where your risk of flare may be higher:

1. If you have PMR and you have swelling and pain of the small joints in your hands and feet, then you may have *polymyalgic-onset rheumatoid arthritis*, or *late onset rheumatoid arthritis*. Alternatively, you may have a form of PMR, but one that tends to run a more chronic course with more flares. Either way, your GP should really refer you to rheumatology (via the local early inflammatory arthritis pathway if one is available) so the diagnosis can be investigated. Additional treatments early on, such as methotrexate, may help reduce the risk of PMR flares, and there is really strong evidence that drugs like this make a big difference if you are found to have rheumatoid arthritis.

2. If you have GCA with evidence of large vessel involvement on scans such as ultrasound, MRI or CT-PET. In that case, you are more likely to have relapsing GCA, so the rheumatologist may also start methotrexate or other DMARDs early on to reduce this risk.

Here is some pragmatic advice, maybe not doctor convention, but distilled from the experiences of hundreds of PMR and GCA sufferers, offered in HealthUnlocked FAQs:

> *"A flare happens when you've gone below the level of pred your illness requires. Either you have reduced too low or you are too active for your medication to control the illness. Sometimes a return to the previous dose is enough, but if it's got too bad it's recommended to add 5mg to the dose at which you last felt all right. Stay there for 7-14 days and then drop down to just above the dose you flared at. You are not reducing relentlessly to zero [although the plan of course for most of us is to get there in the end] - you are looking for the lowest dose that gives the same result as the starting dose did when you first went onto steroids."*

You might ask who is recommending patients to add 5mg to the dose at which they last felt OK, and this would be a good question. This is perhaps the subject over which doctors' and patients' perspectives vary the most. When does a pragmatic approach to varying your dose spill over into self-medicating? Over the years patient wisdom has grown and the moderators on the PMRGCAuk online forum have developed a lot of knowledge from the experience of literally thousands of members. Before experimenting with your dose, though, do talk things over with your doctor. There might be strong medical reasons why you shouldn't adjust your steroid taper on your own initiative.

Here are Vanessa's suggestions for how you might steer that conversation with your doctor to make sure you are covering all the bases.

Vanessa says: on discussing dose adjustment with your doctor

If an element of self-management of your taper is resisted by your doctor, then consider saying this...

"Of course, Doctor, I don't want to be on more steroid than I need, but adequate control of my PMR/GCA is of most importance to me and I would like to receive the dose needed to keep my PMR/GCA under control and to allow me to recover from being on long term steroids. I understand this will vary from person to person because these are often relapsing illnesses with no fixed time frame. I recognise this may slow my taper and put me at higher risk of steroid side effects, so please can we look at managing those potential side effects too?

I'm already on bone and stomach protection; can we look at "steroid protection" in general? Is my blood pressure OK? What is my HbA1c? [a marker of sugar levels over the previous couple of months]. Can I have my cholesterol checked? I'm minimising all my cardiovascular risk factors: I don't smoke and I'm doing my best with my weight and exercise. I've been to the opticians, and my cataracts are stable and my eye pressures are OK. Can we meet in due course to check if everything is still on track?

I understand that you may be worried about my other health problems. So please can we also think about how to manage other things like osteoarthritis (can we look at my pain killers and would a physio referral help?) or (on lower doses) might there be some adrenal suppression causing symptoms?"

If you notice steroid withdrawal symptoms after every dose drop, then also discuss that.

This process may reassure your doctor that, together, you are doing everything to get your risk benefit balance of steroids right, and this is being monitored by you between appointments. The discussion might also help you to understand why your doctor is more reticent if some of these areas are less well controlled.

---- x ----

I have PMR – should I see a rheumatologist?

When a patient with PMR finds that the taper experience is bumpy and spiky and not going very well, perhaps with multiple flares, they may well feel they would benefit from a referral to a hospital specialist. Whether or not you feel this would be right for you will depend on several factors, including your relationship with your GP, and how well your GP knows you, as well as the closeness of the area rheumatologist service and whether there is anyone there who takes a particular interest in PMR. It is worth taking a look at the website of your local hospital trust and navigating to 'R' for Rheumatology in the list of services. Quite often there is a 'meet the team' section with biographies of consultants, which can tell you whether there is a PMR or GCA specialist inhouse. If you can't find this information though, don't be disheartened - any consultant rheumatologist will be able to see and help you.

You need to be clearheaded, well-informed, and prepared to make your case with your GP if you really think you could benefit from a consultation. Spend some time planning and thinking through what you want from a rheumatology consultation and how to convince your GP.

Are you in one or more of the groups where referral is recommended somewhere in your PMR journey? Here is a list of such groups, distilled from the 2010 BSR PMR Guidelines, and the NICE Clinical Knowledge Summary on PMR:

- Age less than 55 years.
- Chronic onset (more than two months). Symptoms have built up slowly and gradually over time, rather than being sudden.
- Lack of shoulder involvement, i.e. no pain or stiffness in the shoulders.
- Absence of inflammatory stiffness. Typically, this kind of stiffness is worse in the morning and eases with gentle movement.
- Prominent systemic features, weight loss, night pain, weakness worse than pain and stiffness, tingling, numbness. These symptoms might be suggesting an alternative cause.
- Features of other rheumatic disease, e.g. swelling in the wrists and hands might suggest rheumatoid arthritis, or tell-tale cranial symptoms that might suggest GCA. In these cases, your GP might be able to refer you quickly to the local Early Inflammatory Arthritis service, or the GCA fast-track service.
- Normal inflammatory markers. Generally, some abnormal inflammation would be expected.
- Higher than typical (for PMR) inflammatory markers – might this be a normal inflammatory response by the immune system against an injury or infection?
- The person is at high risk of adverse effects from steroids.
- Impossible to reduce steroids at intervals without flare.
- Significant steroid side effects.
- The need for prolonged steroid therapy (more than two years).

People with GCA will already be "under" a consultant rheumatologist who is overlooking their ongoing treatment and progress.

I asked Vanessa to give us lay people an insight into what might be going through a rheumatologist's mind when they first meet a PMR referral patient, and her response is presented in the following section.

Vanessa says: on meeting your rheumatologist for the first time

When the rheumatologist sees you, they will assess you to convince themselves that the PMR symptoms are typical, then seek out any features that might suggest a "PMR-mimic" and do extra tests.

The main mimics to exclude are various kinds of arthritis. There are no less than 100 kinds of arthritis, although about 10 types make up most cases. They may do tests focused on joints of the arms and legs if it sounds like rheumatoid, psoriatic arthritis or a crystal arthritis like pseudogout. These might include extra blood tests, as well as X-rays or ultrasound. We may look for inflammatory spine disease, called spondyloarthropathy with blood tests and MRI scans. But often it's osteoarthritis that is contributing to symptoms at least in part. We will also consider if it might be GCA, based on your 'story', and may arrange extra tests for that.

Something in your story might alert us to rarer things like some forms of vasculitis or a connective tissue disorder and then a broader set of tests may be needed.

Sometimes it doesn't appear to be a direct problem of the joints, bones or muscles at all and it's due to a metabolic problem like thyroid disease or low vitamin D, or a nerve related problem. Occasionally we pick up a chronic infection or cancer. And sometimes all the tests are normal, and the person appears to have fibromyalgia, a condition thought to involve abnormal pain processing in the brain, leading to chronic widespread pain, often associated with poor quality sleep and increased sensitivity to touch. You can get fibromyalgia on its own, or as a result of any chronic pain condition, including PMR.

In my clinic, I will have an especially close look for rheumatoid (why rheumatologists are always examining your hands) and for GCA, as both conditions can start with PMR symptoms.

Sometimes, it's really not clear and we have to make a plan based on what it might be. That will often involve discussions around uncertainty and trying to reduce the prednisolone dose to see if the problem gets clearer on the lower dose.

We only tend to see people down the line once they've been on steroids a while and the underlying problem is masked. This of course is the obvious argument for fast-track PMR clinics where people can be seen by a rheumatologist before steroids are started, although these are generally not available in the NHS.

---- x ----

Of course, you may struggle to get that referral. Your GP may consider it more appropriate for you to get through PMR in primary care[21]. You might find it helpful to print off the latest guidelines from the PMRGCAuk website[13] and take them along to the surgery with you. Keep a detailed diary too, of your daily dose and the symptoms you are experiencing.

How it was for me

Here is my story about trying to wean myself off steroids and my experience of a hospital referral. Bear in mind that this was nearly twenty years ago, but I've heard enough stories from others to reassure me that it's still not atypical. Not everyone finds steroid tapering difficult. My mother found it straightforward to reduce her prednisolone dose according to the doctor's schedule and came off it altogether within two years. I found it much harder. I did eventually manage to come right off. I realise that this might sound incredibly self-satisfied and smug, and I wouldn't blame you at all for thinking 'it's alright for her, she obviously hasn't suffered the way I have.' But I did suffer. I was really unwell a good deal of the time.

A year after diagnosis, my PMR was trundling along, sometimes in the background, sometimes demanding more attention. The doctor had given me a chart showing how to get down to 1mg per day over exactly two years from the 20mg starting dose. There would be little in the way of monitoring my ESR and CRP levels: I should just do the taper regardless.

I got down to 12.5mg per day fairly easily but getting below that was extremely difficult. Pain and illness did not disappear with the steroids. I had night sweats, very disturbed sleep, and pain that would make me cry out in the night. I could not turn over in bed without my husband having to get out of bed, walk round to my side and manhandle me over. My PMR was not well controlled. Because I was in my fifties, everything was complicated by the fact that I was in the last phase of a difficult menopause.

On holiday, the heat seemed to sap the life out of me, and I had no energy left to cope with the pain. I went back to using a walking stick. Only in the sea did I feel restored to my 'real' self. While swimming I had some ease and grace, and with the tepid saltwater holding me up, I felt almost pain-free.

Eventually the GP referred me to the rheumatology department at the local hospital. In three visits, I saw three different doctors. On the second, I did at least have a bone scan. Everything OK there, thank goodness. I was never offered alendronic acid during my treatment, but I would have taken it as a precaution had I been. I was taking my Adcal tablets religiously, especially since my mother had had a series of fractures after having PMR and had been one of the first people in the country to have a shoulder replacement.

On the third hospital visit, two years after diagnosis, I was seen by a Polish locum rheumatologist. I was still on 10mg daily and he was a man on a mission. “You must come off these steroids,” he said, “These steroids are very bad for you. Your body, it loves these steroids!” He acted all shocked that I should be on steroids at all (I have since found out that in Poland, methotrexate is the drug of choice). This shook me up no end. I had been in denial about how ill I was. I knew about the side effects and other risks, but I had not really thought before that my body had a chemical dependence on prednisolone. Was I some kind of addict? He stood behind me and pushed my arms down to test my strength. He told me to resist the force and push upwards. We were almost locked in combat for a few seconds. I felt a strange rush of emotion. This doctor was actually prepared to lay hands on me, human to human.

“You are a very strong woman!” he declared, and put me straight down to 7.5mg, with strict instructions to come off prednisolone completely within three months. I was all fired up. I would do it for him.

A month later, at 5mg, I was back at the GP’s surgery, unable to cope. Dr Bush put me back up to 7.5mg and explained gently that I was getting the worst of both worlds. “What is the point of taking a dose of steroids if it is not enough to deal with the symptoms? You are getting all the risks and none of the benefits.” Instead of helping me recover from the illness, all my life force was going into combating the stiffness and chronic pain. “And chronic pain is the surest road to depression”, he said.

We agreed that I had a problem with trying to be a brave soldier, and that from now on we would manage the PMR together, without the help of the hospital. It took me nearly another two years to come off the steroids altogether. I still do not know whether I did the right thing, but I never went back to the hospital again.

I had adjusted my job demands but still had to work three days a week and look after my grandson another three days a week. I would have two-year old Tom from 8 am, Monday through

Wednesday, and we would pick up his big brother from school and I'd give them tea. Then early on Thursday morning I would travel to Oxford to teach for three days, coming back on Saturday night. I was doing all this at the same time as having a chronic illness. This would mean that I would have a few days of feeling unwell and uncomfortable every time I tried to reduce my dose. But I was prepared to put up with this because I had felt similar the last time I had reduced and found that I didn't need to go back up again.

I was telling myself that this was my pattern, my way of reducing, and I could cope with it. Sometimes it was sheer bloody mindedness that got me through. After months of taking 2.5, then 2, then a single milligram a day, I took the step of alternating a steroid-free day with a day with a 1mg tablet. And eventually I gave up the single tablet. There were months of having occasional "PMR days", but I didn't go back to the steroids, although I kept two blister packs of prednisolone in my bedside table for three years, just in case.

I was very conscious of my age. I was just nudging sixty, and most definitely did not see myself taking prednisolone for the rest of my life. It might have been a very different matter had I been nudging eighty instead. In that case I might well have said "I'll take the side effects (real and potential) because what matters most to me is my quality of life right now."

By the time I was coming off steroids I was also involved with the embryonic charity PMRGCAuk, and meeting a supportive group of researchers and clinicians who were not only interested in PMR and GCA, but invested in improving things for patients. It probably made a psychological difference to me that I had their support. At the same time, I can appreciate that being ill and stuck had driven me to look for a support organisation, and when I hadn't found one, had spurred me on to help get one going.

My symptoms of debilitating pain and malaise in the later stages of tapering were, I understand now, probably signalling steroid withdrawal syndrome[38]. My entire system had adapted to being on steroids and needed to recalibrate to the new dose. Bound up in this, I may also have had some steroid-induced adrenal insufficiency.

When tapering down to very much lower doses, some doctors encourage patients to take a dose every other day, as this might have the effect of helping the adrenal glands to kick back into action. But this isn't advisable until the dose is very low (less than an average of 1mg per day), as it is linked to a higher rate of flare. An alternative might be to cut 1mg pills in half or persuade your doctor to give you the much more expensive half-milligram tablets (good luck with that!). Some people feel that it helps to take part of their dose in the morning and part at night, on the basis that they feel it makes them sleep better and wake up with less stiffness in the morning. But this isn't advised in the guidelines either, because there is a risk that this could increase the chance of adrenal insufficiency.

Cumulative dosage: some calculations

It is obvious that, if you are going to have flares, you will end up taking more steroids than you would have done if you had had a smooth taper. And it is the cumulative dose of steroids, as much the dose at any one time, that has the insidious long-term effect on the body.

The international working group on PMR recognised that doctors are keen to get patients down on their dosage as quickly as possible. In the case of PMR, in an ideal situation, if a patient starting on 15mg gets down to 10mg and then reduces by 1mg per month, their steroid regime will last for just twelve months, and they will take a cumulative dosage of 2475mg over this one-year period. That sounds like a good scenario, but short duration of therapy is associated with relapses, and this is precisely what patients are worried about.

Another scenario is a patient who tries to drop and then yo-yos up and down repeatedly between 7mg and 10mg for a year. They might by the end of that year have taken nearer 4000mg, and still not have got to below 7 mg per day, which might take them another year, or more. Their cumulative dose is probably going to be at least 7000 mg over the course of their illness. And they've had to cope with multiple flares in the process.

A third scenario is the person who gets down to 10mg per day (total weekly dose 70mg) inside two months and then reduces much more slowly by reducing their total weekly dose by only 1mg a week for 70 weeks. They will have been on steroids for 18 months and will have taken during that time 3275mg to get down to zero.

Now, just think that 3275mg is just over 3 grams, which is just over one-tenth of an ounce, taken over a year and a half, you can just see how potent prednisolone is. And yet, we have not had any decent systematic double-blinded study that compares the effectiveness of these different ways of tapering steroids. I don't know about you, but I think a lot of patients would like to see this study being carried out for PMR and for GCA. If we felt there was more concerted effort to help us taper in the most appropriate way, we might be more positive about taking this medication. We could put up with the side effects, if we knew we are suffering as little as possible and not taking more of the medication than we needed.

Once again, we are confronted with the reality that it's not so simple - it's horses for courses, and everyone has to work out what's best for themselves in partnership with their clinicians.

There is one school of thought among patients that it may be OK if you can't get down to zero and end up taking a low daily dose of steroids for the rest of your life. Personally, because of the cumulative dose, I don't share that view, although I sympathise with it. I feel strongly that, if you can get down below five milligrams a day, it would be worth making a big push to come down further. Remember, a majority of patients who have had PMR or GCA do come off steroids altogether, so why should you not be one of them? Give it a go.

Steroid sparing

In the UK, the vast majority of PMR patients and many GCA patients will not be offered any 'steroid sparing' medication until later in their treatment when it becomes apparent that the steroids are not working well or quickly enough. For most people with PMR or GCA, however, prednisolone works on the inflammation. It deals with the symptoms and restores something approaching normal life to the patient. It is an unusually inexpensive drug as well, which is fortunate for the NHS, but perhaps not so fortunate for the patient.

When it comes to steroid therapy for PMR and GCA, one of the problems, paradoxically, is that the medicine is inexpensive. Prednisolone is one of the cheapest drugs available to the health service. To the British National Health Service, a 1 mg or 5mg oral tablet of prednisolone costs less than 5p (that is little more than six cents in US money). 2.5mg oral tablets, 0.5mg tablets, solutions and soluble pred are more expensive. I worked out how much a case of PMR costs the health service in drugs if the patient just takes prednisolone and follows the 'classic' course of starting off on 15mg per day and gradually tapers over a two-year period. The figure I came up with was about £60. That is an average of £30 a year, at 2026 prices.

Now, steroids may be nasty in some ways, but for most cases in PMR and GCA they *work,* at least 'well enough'. Therefore, it is not difficult to see that the economists in the National Health Service are not going to be pushing too hard to pay for an alternative to steroids for everyone. Especially not for treating elderly folks. Call me biased, but I rather think that there would be more clamour to find an alternative if GCA and PMR attacked children.

By the same token, given that Big Pharma (the global pharmaceutical industry) is driven by profit, and not altruism, it's not difficult to see that there isn't a big profit motive in researching alternatives to prednisolone for PMR. For GCA things are changing, but PMR is still lagging behind.

Since the last edition of this book, it is encouraging to see further research into ways of reducing cumulative dose. These treatments are not replacements for steroids, but rather 'steroid-sparing' approaches, combining lower doses of prednisolone with another medication to reduce the overall cumulative dose.

And this is where we turn in the next chapter.

5 Treatment beyond steroids

If you have a straightforward and not-too-severe bout of PMR, or even GCA, you may find you are able to taper down to zero prednisolone in the space of a couple of years. But you will be one of the lucky ones. Evidence is stacking up to confirm that these lucky ones are outnumbered by people who are taking steroids for a good while longer than two years, with the relapsing forms of these conditions.

Can I take painkillers?

Many of us were brought up to be stoical and to avoid painkillers as though there is something morally dubious about them. There is no point in this. As my doctor pointed out that time when he had to give me a particularly strong talking-to, putting up with chronic pain is a sure path to depression. Why use your psychic energy fighting pain when you could be using it to heal yourself?

When I found myself yo-yoing up and down from 7.5mg per day, Madeleine Whitlock, a rheumatology nurse who worked with Professor Dasgupta, reminded me painkillers are allowed. That is paracetamol (Tylenol in US), or for those who can take it without suffering constipation, co-codamol. Non-steroidal anti-inflammatories such as Ibuprofen are not effective as the main treatment for PMR or GCA and should not be used instead of steroids.

But taking a maximum of 8 paracetamol a day (four doses of two 500 mg tablets), should not hurt you, unless you are frail, even if you take it every day for a couple of weeks. Do discuss this with your doctor, especially if you have, or have had, any liver or kidney problems. For most people the recommended dose is within safe limits. I found if I took a couple on waking up, I could sometimes make it to about three o'clock in the afternoon before I started to feel the pain too much again. From that conversation on, every time I reduced my dose of pred, I would take paracetamol every day for a few days and give my body a chance to adapt to the lower dose.

Aspirin and statins

Some of you with GCA may have been prescribed a low-dose ("baby") aspirin. This was included in older BSR guidance but has been removed from more recent recommendations because the evidence for benefit is limited. Aspirin and statins are sometimes considered in GCA because of their effects on blood vessels. Aspirin may help to reduce clot formation in inflamed, narrowed arteries, which could in theory lower the risk of complications such as vision loss, but this needs to be balanced against the risk of bleeding.

Many of us older folk are taking statins. Statins may also have anti-inflammatory effects and may be helpful for general vascular health. However, the evidence for benefit in GCA is limited and mixed. So neither is routinely recommended specifically for treating GCA. Instead, they are considered on a case-by-case basis.

In PMR, there is even less evidence of any direct benefit, and these treatments are usually prescribed only for standard cardiovascular reasons rather than for GCA or PMR themselves.

Alternatives to steroids?

There is no doubt the medical world is waking up to the need to find alternatives to steroids for PMR and GCA[39,40,41].

Many patients too would love to see a viable, safe and affordable substitute for prednisolone. However, there is also evidence many people have a more nuanced view of their essential medication.

The international working group for PMR guidelines had to gather data on patients' perceptions of the risks and benefits of medication, compared to the symptoms of the disease. Because we tend to hear a lot about how much people hate the meds, especially steroids, and want to get off them, it would be easy to get the impression that people think of medications as at worst the enemy, at best a necessary evil. There was an interesting result when PMRGCAuk polled members of the HealthUnlocked web forum community about their attitudes to the risk of suffering side effects.

We found the overwhelming majority of voters were on balance positive about their medication. Out of 108 voters, three out of ten agreed strongly with the statement "I would rather take the risks of side effects from medication than lower my quality of life with PMR symptoms". Another 50% of respondents were in general agreement. But around 9% of voters felt the other way – that in some ways the medication is worse than the illness.

Clearly, we have a love-hate relationship with steroids. All the more reason why, personally, I would like to see more doctors prepared to try steroid-sparing drugs (DMARDs) with PMR and GCA, to reduce the patient's overall consumption of prednisolone, as has become commonplace in the treatment of rheumatoid arthritis.

DMARDS

This section looks at this family of drugs known as DMARDs, which stands for disease-modifying antirheumatic drugs.

DMARDs work by suppressing the body's overactive immune and/or inflammatory systems, so PMR and GCA become less active and need less steroid to keep them under control, so they are "steroid sparing". They take effect over weeks or months and are not designed to provide immediate relief of symptoms. There are quite a few different DMARDs, but the most common ones used in PMR and GCA are methotrexate (MTX) and leflunomide (LEF), where either steroids haven't been effective, or the patient has been unable to tolerate them so well. The doctor's decision to offer a DMARD depends on several factors, including the stage and severity of the condition, the balance between possible side effects and expected benefits, and patient preference. Before treatment begins, the patient and clinician should discuss the benefits and risks of each type of therapy, including possible side effects and toxicities, dosing schedule, monitoring frequency, and expected results.

Methotrexate

Methotrexate was originally used as a chemotherapy treatment for cancer. In PMR and GCA, it is used in much smaller doses once a week, but many patients are apprehensive about it. Methotrexate should always be taken alongside folic acid (at least once a week, not on the day you take Methotrexate) to reduce the risk of side effects such as a queasy feeling, upset stomach and a sore mouth. Temporary hair loss is a recognised side effect, but steroids can do this too. MTX is usually prescribed as tablets taken once a week, but you may be offered it as a weekly injection given under the skin using a pre-filled pen device. This reduces the chance of an upset stomach and tiredness and increases the body's uptake of the medication to ensure the full dose is getting to where it's needed. Take it after your evening meal, so you may sleep through these feelings. It's not uncommon to notice a distinct "day-after tiredness", especially early on in treatment. You may have to plan around it and have a quiet next morning, especially for the first few weeks.

Methotrexate can interfere with the bone marrow's production of blood cells, particularly white blood cells called *neutrophils*. When neutrophil levels are low, the risk of infection is increased. Mild drops in neutrophil count may happen in a small number of people. Severe drops (called neutropenia) are rare, usually fewer than 1 in a 100 people. The risk is increased if you have kidney problems and your doctor will give you a lower dose to account for this. Liver toxicity can also occur. Mild, short-term changes in liver blood tests happen in about 15-30 out of every 100 people taking methotrexate. These usually settle down on their own. Ongoing, repeated changes in liver tests happen in about 5 in every 100 people.

Serious liver damage, like scarring (liver fibrosis) or even liver failure (cirrhosis) is very rare, especially if you have blood tests regularly, you take folic acid alongside methotrexate and you limit or avoid alcohol. In fact, people using methotrexate are strongly discouraged from drinking excess alcoholic beverages because of the increased risk of liver damage with this combination. Any potential liver and bone marrow toxicity can be monitored with regular blood tests and the dose adjusted or stopped if this occurs. So, Methotrexate and in fact most DMARDs are safe medications as long as you are prepared to have regular blood tests. Unlike steroids, you can come off MTX immediately without adverse effects if it doesn't suit.

Other DMARDs

Leflunomide, taken by mouth once daily, inhibits production of inflammatory cells. Side effects may include rash, temporary hair loss, liver damage, nausea, diarrhoea, peripheral neuropathy, weight loss, and abdominal pain, plus small blood pressure rises. Like MTX, regular testing to monitor for liver damage and blood abnormalities is required.

Azathioprine (AZA) and Mycophenolate Mofetil (MMF) are other DMARDs used to treat autoimmune and inflammatory diseases and are also widely used to prevent rejection of transplanted organs. In PMR and GCA, AZA and MMF are generally reserved for people who have not responded to, or have been unable to tolerate, MTX or LEF. They are usually taken by mouth once or twice a day.

We know, from the helpline, the forum, and support groups, that many patients are apprehensive about trying DMARDS. We've thus included quite a long section in which Vanessa presents her perspective as a doctor, seeing patients with GCA and the more challenging PMR cases. I have to say, if I had been offered the option, I would have taken MTX without hesitation, knowing I could stop it immediately if it turned out not to be right for me.

Vanessa says: on Methotrexate (MTX) and Leflunomide (LEF) in GCA and PMR, what's the evidence?

Doctors use treatments when there is evidence that they help, and when the benefits outweigh the risks. That sounds simple, but in practice the evidence varies. The strongest proof usually comes from randomised controlled trials (RCTs). However, observational studies following patients receiving routine care, and expert knowledge, are also useful, especially in PMR and GCA where big RCTs are limited.

MTX has had three RCTs in GCA: two American trials didn't show much benefit, but they were small and used low doses, whilst a Spanish trial showed fewer relapses and slightly lower steroid use. When all three were combined in a meta-analysis (161 patients in total), MTX showed a modest improvement, meaning fewer relapses and a lower overall steroid burden (around 850 mg prednisolone less over a year[42]*. Roughly speaking, treating three to four people prevented one flare. These older trials generally used doses now considered low (7.5-15 mg per week) and so may have underestimated the potential benefit of MTX, compared with the 15-25 mg per week we usually use today. More recent real-world studies have shown mixed results for MTX in GCA. However, it is often prescribed to patients with more severe or relapsing disease, which may make it appear less effective than it really is*[43]*.*

Tocilizumab (Toc) is definitely more effective than MTX[44] *(more on this in the next section), but when Toc is unavailable or unsuitable, MTX is still widely used, because MTX may help some patients, especially by reducing relapse risk.*

LEF hasn't had a randomised trial in GCA, but several observational studies have been encouraging. The biggest looked at over 200 patients and found fewer flares and lower steroid use with LEF compared with steroids alone[45]: after nearly two years, the relapse rate in the LEF group was 15%, compared to 45% in the steroid-only group. Smaller studies say much the same. Even though these aren't randomised trials, the evidence is consistent enough that many rheumatologists specialising in GCA feel comfortable using LEF, especially because they have seen it help people reduce their steroid dose, when previously they were unable to do so.

Based on this evidence, UK and European guidelines recommend considering weekly MTX for GCA, particularly for patients at risk of flare or with steroid-related side effects. Guidelines are heavily based on RCTs which is why LEF isn't included. Given that over 50% of GCA patients will relapse and steroid side effects are almost universal, some rheumatologists (me included) offer DMARDs early on, to maximise their steroid sparing effect. The longer you have been on steroids, and the more side effects you have accumulated, the keener your doctor will be for you to consider a DMARD.

In PMR, older trials of MTX were also mixed; some suggested fewer flares and lower steroid needs, others found little difference, again using lower doses. This meant previous guidelines only suggested MTX in certain situations, such as those with recurrent flares or problems with steroids. Then in 2025, the PMR-MODE trial found that 80% of those given MTX 25 mg weekly were in steroid-free remission at one year compared with 46% with placebo (dummy tablet); MTX users also had fewer relapses and stopped steroids more quickly (on average in about 28 weeks) compared with people on placebo (who took on average about 39 weeks)[46]. This suggests clear benefit using adequate modern doses, although the study only involved newly diagnosed patients under ideal conditions, so results might not reflect the reality of people who flare during tapering or struggle with longer-term steroid use. Would these new results make you want to talk to your doctor about MTX for your PMR? LEF in PMR has only small observational studies so far, but results look promising and a proper RCT is underway.

Not everyone gets on well with MTX or LEF, but then again, the majority do. You won't know if the medication suits you unless you try it for a while, and that's part of making a well-informed decision. Plus, if you try it, your doctor won't be upset if you say it's not suiting you. If you are concerned about side effects, then you can always ask to start on a lower dose to make sure you get on with it, then increase to the dose your doctor thinks you need (e.g., LEF can be started at 10mg alternate days).

That said, it's natural to be hesitant about starting a medication that doesn't offer immediate relief. Steroids work quickly, so their effects are obvious. MTX or LEF work in the background, helping to prevent future problems, which makes their benefit harder to notice. Psychologists call this "present bias": we value immediate outcomes more than long-term ones. But if MTX or LEF helps you reduce or avoid higher doses of steroids, it could mean fewer side effects and less medication overall in the long run.

---- x ----

Biologic DMARDs

Today, a new generation of *biologic* medications is transforming the experience of patients with chronic inflammatory diseases. The term "biologic" means that the active component of the medication is produced by living cells which were originally derived from mammals or humans. Think of them as tiny, microscopic factories grown in big bioreactors - no animals or humans are used in the routine production process. The molecules tend to be larger and more difficult to process than conventional chemical drugs, and so they tend to be more expensive. Sometimes, a lot more expensive.

Tocilizumab ("Toc", or "TCZ") is one of these 'biologic' drugs used in the treatment of chronic inflammatory diseases. It blocks the activity of the cytokine IL-6, which plays a central role in driving inflammation. It doesn't carry the burden of side effects and cumulative damage that is the hallmark of long-term therapy with prednisolone.

Toc is however very expensive indeed. Currently, it costs about £6,000 a year to treat a person with GCA, whereas the cost of treating them with steroids is about £30.

Our campaign to get Toc approved by NICE for recalcitrant cases of GCA

Following the initial GiACTA trial of Toc for GCA, there was compelling evidence for rheumatologists to prescribe it for GCA. In many health care systems around the world including those in EU countries, the USA and Canada, Toc can be used for *any* GCA patient where the doctor thinks it is appropriate for no fixed time limit.

For use in the NHS, medications must be approved by the National Institute of Clinical Excellence (NICE), and where they are recommended for a 'new' condition, must be approved for the new use. This involves a lengthy process of examination of the evidence by NICE committee members, and presentations being made by pharmaceutical companies and other interested parties.

I had the privilege of representing PMRGCAuk on the panel of proposers, alongside eminent rheumatologists, ophthalmologists and Roche experts on GCA. We travelled to Manchester several times to put our case, and we pressed it very strongly. Against us, the only argument that really carried weight with the NICE committee was the cost. Unfortunately, the NHS being what it is, the cost argument was consistently the one the panel seemed to want to give most attention to.

I remember there was a certain amount of ageism implicit in the whole process. There were calculations of *QALYs* - quality-adjusted life years - to my mind a rather ham-fisted technique for measuring the benefits of one form of treatment against another. What it boils down to is the idea that a treatment restoring health to a young person and giving them a normal life expectancy at an acceptable level of health and ability, will carry more QALYs than a very expensive treatment for a condition attacking people at an average age of 70-something.

In the world of QALYs, a new drug to reduce the damaging cumulative effects of steroids on older people who repeatedly flare with GCA, was not going to cut the mustard. Especially when Tocilizumab was so expensive. On the proposing side, we stressed the danger of sight loss and damage to bones. The implications were that having to help people adapt to blindness, or lose their mobility due to a fall, would be more expensive than giving people the drug.

Roche claimed there was little evidence that people with GCA would relapse after a course of Toc. It really did seem to be the miracle drug. We had to wait for the panel verdict. In the end, they approved use of Toc for 'recalcitrant' cases of GCA - GCA that was relapsing or "refractory", i.e. cases that refused to get better on prednisolone - for one year and one year only. The implication was the belief, or hope, that the year would be enough[47].

We were both disappointed and relieved at the same time. We accepted it as a compromise position, knowing it was the best we could hope for at that stage. The alternative would have been to lose access to the drug altogether. We hoped against hope Toc would kick the dragon over a cliff and that would be the end of GCA for those lucky patients, with no relapses. We hoped and hoped.

It soon turned out that, even on Toc, between 15% and 20% of patients still experienced some flaring. Of course, this was a major improvement on the 57% who flare on prednisolone alone. And of course, Toc is sparing steroid toxicity for all patients and reducing anxiety about possible sight loss.

There is now plenty of evidence the dragon does rear its head again after the year on Toc is up[48]. Vanessa led a big study of 40 NHS rheumatology centres which showed that up to half of people flare at some point after coming off Toc[49]. We now face a campaign to get Toc approved for longer than a year for GCA, in fact, for indefinite treatment, if needed. We need your help to do it. Please join PMRGCAuk!

We also hope Toc and its biologic cousins might be approved in the NHS for the more difficult cases of PMR, because randomised trials also show that blocking IL-6 can reduce flares and the amount of steroid needed in PMR. In the PMR-SPARE study of newly diagnosed PMR, 63% of people treated with tocilizumab were in remission without steroids at 16 weeks, compared with 12% of those given placebo. In the SEMAPHORE trial of people with PMR who were unable to reduce steroids, the main treatment goal (good disease control while successfully tapering steroids) was achieved by 67% of patients receiving Toc, compared with 31% on placebo, and 49% were able to stop steroids completely by 24 weeks versus 20% on placebo. In the SAPHYR trial, people with relapsing PMR treated with sarilumab (another IL-6 blocker) achieved sustained remission more often (28% compared with 10%), despite following a much faster steroid-reduction plan.

Sarilumab is licensed for PMR in the States. We are a long way from routine use in the NHS. But patient advocacy is having an influence, as is a new generation of rheumatologists who are excited at the prospect of bringing new drugs to bear on PMR and GCA, even at "first line", when cases are newly diagnosed, just as they can be in other countries.

Vanessa says: on discussing Toc with your doctor

Your question: Am I a candidate for Tocilizumab (Toc or TCZ)?

You may be a candidate if your GCA has flared or isn't responding well to steroids. It is not available for new onset GCA on the NHS. You don't need to have had multiple flares, and you don't need to have tried the more established steroid-sparing agents like methotrexate or leflunomide. If you have significant risks from long-term steroid use (like diabetes, osteoporosis, or previous fractures), then your rheumatologist will be able to argue your case more strongly, but steroid side effects on their own are not a reason to get Toc on the NHS. Of course, if you are struggling, your doctor may recommend a lower or faster steroid taper, which is more likely to lead to flare, reassured that they can reach for Toc if that happens.

What are the pros and cons of tocilizumab?

Pros include better disease control, fewer flares, and reduced steroid. In the landmark GiACTA trial, 56% of patients in the Toc group with a 26-week steroid taper were in sustained remission, compared to just 18% of those without Toc given a 52-week steroid taper. Plus, those on Toc needed half the cumulative steroid dose compared to those without Toc. Cons include that it is only available by injection using a pen device, the risk of tocilizumab side effects, and the possibility it may not work for you. Common side effects of tocilizumab include a higher risk of infections, headaches, raised cholesterol and liver enzymes, and occasionally reduced white blood cell counts. Regular blood tests monitor safety. Bowel perforation is a very rare side effect and those that have had diverticulitis should not have Toc unless there are no alternatives.

What will happen to my steroid taper once I'm on Toc?

Often, the taper speed can be doubled. Imagine you are on 40mg prednisolone daily. When you are just on steroids, rheumatology guidelines suggest reducing by 5mg per week down to 20mg, then by 2.5mg every 2-4 weeks down to 10mg, then by 1mg per month. On Toc, you can potentially reduce by 5mg every 3-4 days down to 20mg, then by 2.5mg every 1-2 weeks down to 10mg, then by 1mg per fortnight. However, steroid withdrawal syndrome and/or steroid-induced adrenal suppression symptoms may mean you can't go that fast, even if your GCA is under good control, so you should discuss your own taper with your rheumatologist, especially when you get to doses less than 10mg daily.

What monitoring is required?

You'll need blood tests every few months to check liver function, white blood cell counts, and cholesterol.

How long would I be on it?

In the NHS in England, treatment is limited to 12 months (watch this space, we hope this will change in the next year or two). Some patients in countries with less restricted access may need longer or repeated courses depending on how their disease behaves after stopping.

What signs should I look out for that might suggest side effects or flare?

Watch for signs of infection (such as fever, cough, or urinary symptoms), abdominal pain (which could suggest bowel issues), or a return of GCA symptoms like headache, jaw pain, or PMR, especially since blood tests may not clearly indicate a flare (CRP and ESR bloods are usually normal on Toc, even when someone is flaring).

Toc is by far the most effective steroid sparing medication available for GCA, so why is my doctor reticent about me having it?

If you don't have a "secure" diagnosis of GCA (one confirmed on imaging such as ultrasound, or by temporal artery biopsy) then it will be much harder for your doctor to argue your case to the GCA funding panel for Toc in your region, unless you have unfortunately had severe complications of GCA such as sight loss. This is not an absolute block to Toc, because during the Covid-19 pandemic several patients complained that they couldn't have the tests because of lockdown. Therefore, if you are in an area where these tests are difficult to access, your doctor might be able to argue your case without them. Because tocilizumab lowers CRP and ESR, making disease activity harder to track, clinicians may be cautious and want strong diagnostic confidence before starting it.

Sometimes your doctor may doubt your symptoms are due to GCA flare, even if you have had a definite diagnosis of GCA in the past. There are also human factors: many doctors trained in the pre-tocilizumab era, when steroids were the only option. It takes time for treatment culture to shift. Some adopt new therapies early; some wait until there is much more evidence from long term studies.

So, the hesitation from your doctor often doesn't mean: "You don't need this." It usually means: "I have to satisfy several clinical and bureaucratic criteria before I'm allowed to give it to you, and I must be certain we'll still be able to safely monitor you once we do". This is not you versus the doctor. It's you and the doctor navigating NHS policy together. The more the discussion focuses on your risk of steroid side effects, your flare history, and GCA disease activity, the more straightforward the conversation should become. Asking your doctor a question like this might be helpful: "Based on how things have progressed so far with my GCA, do you think we're at the point where a funding request for tocilizumab could be considered? And if not yet, what clinical milestones would need to happen before it would be appropriate?"

---- x ----

Patient experiences of being on Tocilizumab

I asked on the web forum for stories from patients who have experience of Toc. It might seem challenging because you have to inject yourself subcutaneously, usually using an auto-injector pen device. Jeff, in the US, wrote to me about his 9-month experience of self-injection with Tocilizumab (marketed as Actemra) for GCA:

> *"The injections are now very routine. I developed a good habit beginning with the first injection. I send myself an email with the time, the location of the injection on my body, and anything unusual of note. This email is like a lab note. It verifies I took the injection. It also allows me to reliably vary the location of the injections on my body.*
>
> *"I am still taking weekly Actemra injections. I have not had any side effects, and they have allowed me to taper the prednisone to 4 mg per day. I am looking forward to the time when I no longer need to take prednisone."*

Lil, in Canada, says:

> *"My Rheumy encouraged me to research the disease and after the biopsy and PET scan, which were positive for GCA, we met and I asked for Actemra [Toc]. My doctor had to*

apply to my government plan for coverage. At the time he said Actemra would "kick prednisone's butt to work faster."

"I'm fortunate that I did not have any side effects with Toc. The only problem I had was that the Doctor had ordered the syringe type which I just couldn't handle so I requested the ACT pen. Other than occasional bruising all is well.

"I wouldn't like to imagine what life would have been like with prednisone only. We all know those side effects. So, I am a big believer in what Actemra can do for patients."

PMRpro, a mainstay of the PMRGCAuk HealthUnlocked patient forum, is one of the few people to have been prescribed Toc for polymyalgia rheumatica. Her story with PMR has been long, over 20 years, because she is one of those people for whom PMR has never gone away. She currently lives in Italy and has a good longstanding relationship with her rheumatologist, who is a specialist in PMR. She says:

"A few months after my husband's death, I had a massive flare - the dose I required to function crept up until I was heading for 20mg. My rheumatologist had tried MTX some years before, but it made me so ill in the first month we discontinued it. So, he went straight to TCZ. There are no time restrictions here....

"It took me about 6 months to taper to 10mg (prednisolone) with no problems at all and I finally got to 6mg. At 6mg I can feel adrenal wobbles with any more than daily tasks - doing the tax returns or dealing with the Italian pension authorities for example! At 5mg daily functioning was hard. I am absolutely stable at 2-weekly injections and 7mg pred. I do notice I am a bit stiffer in the last couple of days before the next injection is due.

"The injection is absolutely no problem for me though I can imagine for some it may feel a bit daunting. I have had no adverse effects with TCZ - not even injection site irritation. I have been on it for over 3 years now - the best thing that has happened to me in 20 years of PMR."

Julianne recently sent me the story of her rollercoaster ride with prednisone and Toc:

"I'm in Australia where Tocilizumab is only available for a year. After my 12 months I reached out to Roche privately and they agreed to subsidise me with the support of my Rheumatologist, and so I was on it for over 3 years.

"Diagnosed with PMR in late 2018, I was unable to taper below 15mg and after a prolonged period of increased CRP and ESR, my Rheumatologist ordered a PET-CT. I had had PMR for 18 months and, the raised markers were diagnosed as GCA/LVV which was evident through the PET.

"I was put on Toc and began a slow taper of prednisolone to zero over a 12- month period. It was I who insisted on the slow taper, being cautious after a couple of previous flares prior to LVV diagnosis. Because Toc caused low neutrophils [white blood cells], my weekly jabs had been spread to fortnightly and eventually to 3-weekly, evidently still doing the job.

"After just over 12 months pred-free, my Rheumatologist asked me to begin a Toc taper and so I reduced to 4-weekly jabs. I had an appointment to see her after several months and just prior, I had the usual blood tests I had discontinued over the previous 12 months. This is when things went awry. My markers had risen to very high levels, and I was put on 25 mg of prednisolone and back to weekly TCZ until my neutrophils began to drop again, so fortnightly jabs.

> *"I managed to taper the prednisolone down to 5mg, but my neutrophils were still playing games and so I came off Toc altogether and ping, up went my CRP and ESR again. So back up to 25mg of pred and another slow taper, without the help of Toc."*

We've quoted these stories at length to show how a pattern emerges. They also illustrate what treatment options may be available to patients outside the UK. They don't completely reflect current practice within the UK, but it's good to have the comparison, and, if you're not in Britain, then do explore all the options available to you.

Toc really does make a difference to people who would otherwise be on very high cumulative doses of steroids over time. However, once the Toc is discontinued, the chances are that in up to half of people, symptoms will return, usually within six months to a year of stopping. We can say it's a fantastic treatment, but not a miracle cure, and the twelve-month rule really needs to be revisited. There are trials looking at reduced dose Toc after the year is up (termed "tapered dose"), and trials looking at whether MTX helps maintain the remission induced by a year of Toc. The evidence of benefit of more than one year of Toc is from increasing numbers of observational trials all over the world, on patients being treated in routine practice.

Other biologics

It's worth bearing in mind that new biologic drugs are continually being developed, trialled, and coming onto the market. They tend to be approved for certain conditions and then, when their efficacy is proven in use, clinicians start to campaign for trials with other conditions.

One such biologic, Sarilumab (marketed as Kevzara), is approved by the Food and Drug Administration (FDA) in the United States for use with PMR. It comes in a self-injection form for use every two weeks. It also blocks IL-6.

Another, rejoicing in the name of Upadacitinib (UPA), is causing some excitement in the rheumatology world. At the time of writing (mid-2026), it has just received approval by the FDA in the United States for use in GCA based on evidence from the SELECT-GCA trial. This showed that it reduced flares and steroid requirements broadly consistent with the kind of improvements seen in the GiACTA trial that tested Toc in GCA. It all takes time, but who knows, by the time you are reading this it may have been approved by NICE. Yet, just as with Toc several years ago, PMRGCauk and other advocates are experiencing a tough battle to get it approved.

By now you will have ample indication that the course of your PMR and GCA may be anything but smooth. A generation of rheumatologists and general practitioners were trained that PMR and GCA are self-limiting diseases that burn themselves out after a couple of years or so. This led to the incorporation in treatment guidelines of medication schedules leading to zero medication after two years. As patients we might see both the logic, since doctors want patients to be off medication as soon as possible, and also the contradiction, because ever since patients have been able to get together to share their experiences it has been self-evident to us that two years was impossibly optimistic for many people. This is not to deny there are people who recover completely within two years. If you're lucky, you will be one of them. But given that both GCA and PMR are flaring diseases, we have to recognise the guidelines are often describing an ideal situation, the situation doctors would want to be the case, and not how it is for perhaps most people.

A response to this contradiction is the concept of "Treat to target", described in a paper from 2024 by a large international multidisciplinary group, including a British patient representative, Lorna Neil[50]. The paper (key points are reproduced in Appendix C at the end of the book) represents a move away from the idea that the object of treatment is to get people off medication. Rather, a treatment plan should be agreed between the clinician and the patient themselves, depending on the goals of the individual, regarding quality of life, risk of relapse, managing other conditions, etc. The group recommended the treatment target for PMR, GCA, and cases of both PMR and GCA concurrently, should be remission: remission being the absence of symptoms and systemic inflammation. Another target for GCA is the avoidance of vascular damage. The group recognised medication should be at an appropriate level to maintain remission, and that drug-free remission may be achieved in a proportion of cases.

This is a major step forward, not only from the point of view of treatment and medication plans going forward, but also from the psychological point of view for patients. No longer should anyone who doesn't manage to get fully off medication feel they are failing in some way, that they are not good patients, or there is something lacking in the way they have been managing their own condition.

We are some way off from understanding precisely what is the difference in the disease mechanisms between "simple" PMR, that self-limits and enables you to recover completely, and "refractory" PMR, which requires you to continue with a low level of medication indefinitely. However, I count it as progress that doctors all around the world are acknowledging that PMR and GCA are a tad more complicated than they were once made out to be, and patients who don't manage to get off medication are not atypical but a different kind of typical.

In this chapter we've looked at current and future medications that promise to reduce the overall burden of reliance on steroids and help you get better, should your dragon be particularly troublesome. In the next chapter we have a look at things you can do yourself to make things easier.

6 Helping yourself to recovery

This chapter is about what we can do, besides taking our medication, to help ourselves get through the months leading to recovery. It deals with managing pain, work, nutrition and our psychological well-being.

As you read through it and think about what you might choose to put into action or not, a certain amount of self-knowledge will be a great advantage, and I'm sure by now you have plenty of that. What kind of action do you tend to think has most impact on your health and well-being? Are you a person who feels good with lots of exercise, or is your attitude that exercise is a necessary evil? Do you find it easy to control what you eat and drink? Do you use foodie treats to reward yourself for a job well done or to help you get through difficulties? Be honest with yourself about what will suit you and what won't. Don't try to become a different sort of person. You already have enough on your plate with this illness. My advice would be - don't make life harder for yourself than it already is.

What caused my PMR or GCA?

One of the things lots of people beat themselves up about is figuring out what made them fall ill with PMR or GCA in the first place. A study of PMR patients being cared for by their GPs, known as the PMR Primary Care Cohort Study[51], asked patients what they thought might have caused their PMR. This might seem a silly question seeing as it's still a scientific mystery what causes PMR. So why would you ask patients? The point of the question was that it's human nature to try to assign causality to things that happen to us. It helps us come to terms with things, explain them to ourselves and others, and eventually find some closure. It's useful information for doctors because it helps to inform conversations and might even give some indication as to why patients view medication and other treatments cautiously. For example, a patient who is convinced an illness was caused by a poor diet might put more faith in dietary changes than in medication.

Well, it might not surprise you to hear almost half of the cohort answered "No idea" to this question. Some put it down to ageing, nothing more specific than that, others to injury and other forms of strain and stress. The older the respondent, the more likely they were to state age and normal wear and tear as the cause of their PMR. The younger they were, the more likely to cite causes related to work[52].

The story I told myself was of a viral infection, that bout of pneumonia, sending my immune system into overdrive. I understood, in a healthy person, the immune system creates inflammation in the effort to deal with infection or injury. In my story about PMR it became important to me that it is an auto-immune disease, and I should give some attention to calming my immune system down. There was new research revealing the inflammatory chemical IL-6 is much higher in PMR and GCA patients than normal, and even higher than in other inflammatory illnesses such as RA.

This got considerable attention in the second edition of this book, to the point that a couple of rheumatologists suggested I may have over-egged the auto-immune pudding. However, Vanessa agrees that PMR and GCA happen when the immune system becomes overactive and causes inflammation, likely triggered by a mix of age, genetic factors and environmental triggers such as infections.

The infections most often suggested are common viral illnesses such as shingles, parvovirus and flu, but no single infection has been proven to cause PMR or GCA. Many patients report a recent infection before symptoms start, and there is some evidence of seasonal patterns, with more cases seen at certain times of year. Taken together, this suggests infections may act as a trigger in susceptible people, rather than a direct cause.

Had I told myself a different story, my attitude towards my fight with my personal dragon might have been different.

So, take a few moments to ask yourself whether you are telling yourself a story of what caused your PMR and GCA, and then ask whether it's affecting how you view the condition. How do you feel about it emotionally? Are you angry? If yes, who are you angry with? Are you sad because of what you are missing or the things you can't do? Are you accepting and matter of fact about it?

If you're blaming yourself, let yourself off the hook. There is nothing to be gained by punishing yourself. And there is probably nothing you could have done to stop this happening to you.

Will I need to change my lifestyle?

Whatever our stage in life, whether we are at the peak of our career or just embarking on retirement, clearing out the empty nest or caring for aged parents, getting a diagnosis of a chronic health condition is bound to be unsettling. Many people wonder how much their daily and weekly routines are going to change, and whether they will be able to carry on doing the things they were doing perfectly well before. But don't forget many of us let modern life run away with us until our bodies yell "Enough!"

Can I exercise like before? Can I carry on with my high-powered job? Will I be able to look after my ailing husband? Will I be able to visit my son in Australia? The answer to these questions is always 'It depends'. It depends on your general level of fitness, on your circumstances and the support around you, and, perhaps most of all, on the demands you place on yourself. At the start of your story with GCA and/or PMR, you will be in an acute state of ill-health. You may be feeling pretty rough, so rough in fact that the diagnosis comes as a relief. The steroids may help a lot with this acute phase. But as you start to regain your mobility and feel more like your former self, it can be tempting to throw yourself back into your old routine. This would be a mistake.

Nobody wants you to set up camp on the sofa and not move for two years, but you will need to build rest into your daily and weekly schedule. Only you can work out your optimum level of activity to maximise your wellbeing while not wearing yourself out. Vanessa suggests that aiming for around 50% of your previous level is a reasonable starting point, although you may need to work up to that.

Coping with Pain

We have different responses to pain. In two individuals, the pain threshold and pain tolerance levels may be quite different. The pain threshold is the point at which pain starts to be felt. The level of pain tolerance is the point at which the intensity of pain becomes too much for the person experiencing it.

There is some evidence that men and women might differ when it comes to experiencing and reporting pain. Researchers claim women (in general) seem to feel pain at lower thresholds than men and have lower tolerance levels[53] (I realise many female readers will have a problem believing this!). There are various theories about why this may be the case. It may have something to do with women's emotionality, such as they may tune in to the negative feelings associated with pain more easily, or earlier, than men (in general) do.

Personally, I find this theory unconvincing given the number of women I have known who just get on with life while suffering conditions inflicting chronic pain for years on end. An alternative theory is that women's caring roles mean they are biologically programmed to notice pain in themselves in case this signals an inability to care for other people. A third idea suggests women's apparent increased sensitivity to pain links to levels of hormones in their bloodstreams. Whatever the truth of all this, it is quite evident that being in chronic pain can sap anyone's energy, leading to low mood and even clinical depression.

Lynda wrote to me vividly about her early days of coming to terms with her diagnosis:

> *"Week one I mistrusted the diagnosis. Week 2 I took steroids as a diagnostic. Week 3 I felt better, week 4 I mistrusted the diagnosis and felt very depressed and refused steroids, week 5 I had pain even worse than when I had seen my GP, week 6 had to accept the inevitable, week 7 read everything and hated the meds, week 8 finally had to get on with it. I'm ongoing now on 10mg and feeling some days ok and some days very low. Some days pain, some days mild pain. Strangely, some weeks I look after myself really well and think I am going to be the healthiest person to help me recover then bang - I go into what's-the-point mode and crash both mentally and don't care. I suppose before I had PMR I didn't have to question what's happening today with my body. However, it has made me more empathetic to others who have had years of debilitating illness who can still keep a positive mindset. My aim is to achieve an acceptance and start living the new me positively."*

My own experience with PMR was that, apart from the first couple of days on 20mg of pred, I never had a day without pain. Pain and stiffness went hand-in-hand for me. They were the two sides of the same coin. Sometimes pain caused me more anguish, sometimes stiffness. Eventually I understood I had to come to terms with my pain, almost make friends with it, in order to carry on.

I hear you groan. How can you make friends with your pain? Well, I understood it was not going to go away for a long time, and my pain and I were on a journey together. Like any travelling companion, I could pay attention to it all the time, or not. I could use mindfulness techniques to really concentrate on my pain, to 'get in touch with it'; and in doing so, I realised, although it was very unpleasant, the pain of PMR was not going to destroy me. I am not talking here about the pain of acute GCA, which is a different matter altogether, by the way.

Most mornings, having paid some attention to the pain, and taken a couple of paracetamols with my breakfast, I found there were times when I could become unaware of it, although it was still there. The worst times for me were at night, when I would cry out in my sleep with pain. Had I known then that the levels of IL-6 were highest in my bloodstream in the small hours, I would have asked my doctor about experimenting with taking some of my steroids at bedtime. It might have worsened sleep, but on the other hand my sleep was being disturbed anyway. And note that I would have discussed it with my doctor before experimenting! Here's a caveat from Vanessa.

Vanessa says: on splitting your dose

Whilst there might be some benefits from splitting the dose, there are also potential risks. Taking some of your dose at bedtime might reduce waking with pain or stiffness and might improve sleep disturbed by inflammatory pain, but steroids taken later in the day can worsen insomnia, restlessness and vivid dreams and may also worsen adrenal suppression making steroid tapering harder. Plus, you will be taking a smaller dose in the morning, so it might make things worse in the day. There is very little good research on splitting the dose so it's hard to give good advice on this one. This is definitely one to discuss with your doctor. I don't generally split the dose. Rather I will run through this checklist: Is the illness fully controlled? Is it true disease activity, or steroid withdrawal/adrenal suppression symptoms, or mechanical pain, sleep or mood problems? Is the total daily dose already too low, have the steroids just been reduced too quickly?

---- *x* ----

You may find using a TENS machine is helpful when the pain is particularly bothersome. TENS stands for "transcutaneous electrical nerve stimulation" and works by attaching a couple of pads to the skin and stimulating the nerves by passing a small electric impulse to the affected parts of the body. I did find it worked for me to some extent, but I could never figure out whether it was actually reducing my level of pain, or whether the involuntary contractions of my muscles were just giving me some distraction. Either way, if it helps, what's not to like?

For me, meditation was and is a boon. I no longer have the pain and stiffness of PMR, but I still find myself getting very tense and achy at times, and a few minutes' relaxed meditation gets me back onto an even keel. There is nothing weird about meditation. It is a simple technique for stilling my over-active mind and relaxing the body. There are lots of apps available to help, and you can have fun trying them out.

Work

One of the hardest aspects of living with PMR was coming to terms with its impact on my working life. To begin with, as a university teacher managing a large department in a business school, I did not have time to be ill. Over a period of three months, I had gone from running at least ten miles a week, to walking with a stick, and being almost unable to haul myself out of bed. Once diagnosed, I thought back and realised I had probably been feeling unwell for some time and had had a constant headache for weeks; but I kept putting it down to the stress of my busy and high-pressured job. I went for weeks and weeks ignoring the worsening stiffness in my shoulders, putting it down to tension. On one level, I knew I was ill, but my attention was elsewhere, until I simply could not go on any longer and my body called time on me.

At 54, I was young to get polymyalgia rheumatica, and I quickly discovered PMR and GCA do not appear on the radar of most employing organisations. Because they are regarded as illnesses of the elderly there has been little research on the impact having PMR or GCA has on a person's working life. Certainly, there are worse things that can go wrong with us in middle age than getting polymyalgia rheumatica, or even GCA. But these illnesses are so little known and so poorly understood, people who do get them are at a real disadvantage when it comes to working out how they are going to affect them at work.

Once the steroids performed their magic and I was able to carry on working, I tried to carry on as if nothing was wrong. There was a huge physical and mental effort involved. I would have to get up in the middle of a meeting to walk around the table and stretch my crooked body out. I was not such a good listener to my colleagues and students, because the amount of physical discomfort I was in was sapping my attention. I was becoming a grumpy old woman.

After a few months, I realised I would have to scale down and took a job at a new place at a lower level on the career ladder. After a few months in this new job, I went part-time. I was filling up the rest of the week with childcare, which was a joy, but demanding in its own way. I was definitely asking too much of my body, and my mind, to be honest.

Nevertheless, I did feel much better, but I had to come to terms with the fact this was going to affect me for the rest of my life, because it would hit my income forever. My earnings had dropped. My pension would be less. PMR started a process of gradual disengagement from my punishing career as a senior academic, which undoubtedly cost me a six-figure sum in the ten years between the ages of 55 and 65. Then there was the loss in status. It took me a while to let go of my career as something that mattered to me more than my health. There was some grieving to do. Still, I was one of the lucky ones – I was able to carry on working.

Many people have a much worse time than me. If you're a builder and you can't climb a ladder or lift a heavy weight, what are you going to do? What if your livelihood depends on you driving your van, and you've lost the sight in one eye? Yes, I know in theory you can drive with monocular vision, and some do, but on today's roads? I wouldn't like the prospect myself.

Let's hear from a few people who have kindly offered to share their stories, starting with Heather, a primary school teacher:

> *"As a nursery class teacher working in a primary school, the physical side of my job became increasingly more unmanageable. At first, it was just difficulty getting up off the floor after an activity with a group of children, but then I seemed to lose muscle strength and stamina, making simple physical tasks extremely challenging for me.*
>
> *"Lifting resources and equipment up & down onto & off shelves, was completely exhausting, and over time I was achieving less and less. Eventually the fatigue was too much and when every day felt like an endurance test, I knew I had to take some sick leave.*
>
> *"School literally did everything they could to facilitate my return to work, but the demands of a class of 26 four-year-olds was simply too much.*
>
> *"I made two further attempts at returning to work, but both were unsuccessful. On each return, I'd felt ready to go back, but within four weeks, I was struggling with the extreme fatigue again. Eventually, I was medically retired.*
>
> *"Although I was devastated to leave the job I adored, in some ways, it was a blessing. It meant that I had the time and space I needed to rest, and the stress & pressure from not knowing if I'd be well enough for work each morning, was completely removed."*

Here is 'Alec', a former architect, talking about one of the most difficult cognitive effects of long-term medication for a professional person:

> *"I have given up my professional practice after realising I suffer from 'brain-fog' for around 9 months of every year whilst reducing prednisolone dosage and trying new 'helper' drugs every year. I was finally prescribed a tocilizumab 162mg/week pen in 2025. My brain can now focus but aches continue below 8mg/day prednisolone. I may return to property development but have deregistered as an architect as I consider myself unsafe to practise with brain-fog (and I've reached state pension age). I'm continuing with a reduced level of voluntary work as a council member of a learned society, having dropped out or failed to be appointed for other voluntary posts due to ...brain-fog."*

Stella, at 71, is retired from paid work, but was continuing to contribute as a writer and researcher until PMR struck. For her the fatigue was one of the hardest things to cope with. She told me about the importance of her work to her sense of identity:

> *"Prior to PMR I had (almost) unlimited mental and physical energy, eager to get up in the mornings and get on with the day. I have always loved my work and had not long retired from paid work. I was diagnosed with PMR in September 2024 (triggered by Covid at the end of June), and prescribed steroids.*
>
> *"As well as being limited physically, I hit a mental 'brick wall'. I found I could not open my computer, read relevant publications, engage with things I cared about or do any 'work'. It felt as though I was burned out and my mind needed to completely disengage. This lasted for about six months, since when I have gradually re-engaged.*

> *"During the brick wall period, I could not have worked at all, and it is still limited. I can concentrate for a couple of hours at a time but am mentally finished by about 6pm. I can't tackle anything in the evening. So, everything takes much longer.*
>
> *"But I am better for working, no matter how little. I enjoy it and it has a purpose. It is my familiar old self, albeit modified."*

It's so important for us, and actually for the whole of society, to realise how important the contribution of retired people is, either as volunteer workers, or carers. Here is Lil, in Canada, underlining that point:

> *"As fatigue has taken over my life, I have even resigned from my volunteer opportunities as I never know from one day to the next whether I will be able to complete any shifts given to me. I keep hoping that someday it will burn itself out."*

In our post-Covid world, so many people are working from home for at least part of the week. We are also online much more and staring at a screen for hours on end. This is enough to stiffen up the supplest of youngsters, so people with musculoskeletal conditions have to be extra-careful.

Let's face it, getting PMR or GCA while you are still of working age is no joke. It has a massive effect on all aspects of your life. Having listened to lots of people now, I would say to anybody 'Don't try to pretend nothing has happened and carry on regardless. If you have help at hand, like an Occupational Health department, use it. A good employer may even be pleased to know about your illness because, as far as they are concerned, if they can help you, it shows they are fulfilling the requirements of disability legislation. I was amazed to find I became a "good" statistic as far as my employer was concerned. It was a relief to come out and admit I needed help to be able to carry on doing my job.

As people's work lives become ever longer, there will be more and more people bringing PMR and GCA to work. However, we have a long way to go before employers really understand the help and support people need when they get PMR or GCA during their working lives.

Housework

Do you find you cannot keep the house as clean and tidy as it used to be? We all know keeping the house nice is not the most important thing in the world. However, it certainly helps, when you are feeling down, to be in a pleasant environment. I asked people with PMR and GCA for their tips on keeping on top of housework rather than letting it get on top of you. Here are their ideas!

a) Keep a small basket at the bottom of the stairs. When you think of something you need to take upstairs, pop it in the basket until you need to go up anyway.

b) Get rid of heavy pottery storage jars (even if they are pretty) and replace them with lightweight plastic or aluminium ones.

c) As soon as you can muster the energy, have a good clear-out. Cut down the amount of clutter in your home merely attracting dust. A good declutter can be fantastically uplifting. If you feel some things have memories for you, take photos of them to keep – the memories will still be there. Make sure you have some help to get unwanted stuff out of the house.

d) Keep a packet or two of surface wipes handy around the house. They really are good at picking up dust and sticky marks. Much less trouble than lugging a bowl of water around.

e) If you have space, keep a second lightweight vacuum cleaner upstairs.

f) Wipe down the tiles in the shower after you have showered, while you're still in the buff. Or clean the bathroom in the nude and then treat yourself to a lovely long soak.

g) Do one room completely, one at a time. Don't try to do more than one room a day. Then, if one room is a mess, you can go into the room you have done and give yourself a big pat on the back (well, metaphorically anyway).

h) Do you have a space upstairs near the bathroom? Plumb the washing machine in upstairs and move the dryer up too if you have one. This is how people in Europe organise things. Take the ironing board and iron upstairs too. Use a spare bedroom as a utility room. Saves lots of trudging up and down stairs with piles of dirty and clean washing. And it keeps it all out of sight.

i) Cut down the amount of bedding you have to wash. Using a top sheet under the duvet cover saves washing the duvet cover too often. When you change the sheets, this top sheet becomes the bottom sheet. This way, you only have to wash one sheet at a time. Don't even think about ironing them!

j) If you have an adult son or daughter, jot down a note of things they can do for you next time they come to see you. Don't feel guilty about asking. They are usually happy to do something for you. It gives them a warm glow.

k) Don't be afraid to ask for help from family and friends. They need to understand you are unwell, even if they think you look marvellous, with your disappearing wrinkles and blooming skin.

Physical activity and exercise

The next chapter is all about physical activity and exercise when you have PMR or GCA. So, we're not covering it in detail here, but it would be remiss of us not to mention it in a chapter on helping yourself, seeing as maintaining our strength and mobility is a key aspect.

Clearly, the issues involved in physical activity and maintaining movement are different if you are 53 or 83 at diagnosis. We all have different starting points. I know many 70-year-olds who are fitter and more energetic than several 40-year-olds of my acquaintance.

Before I became ill with PMR, I was a runner. I had run the London Marathon at the age of 49 and had carried on doing occasional half-marathons. At 54, I was pretty fit. However, PMR put paid to that, and I had to scale down to walking. Once on prednisolone, I could still go on a long walk of about six miles, but I could only do it once a week. It hurt, but it was worth it. I could still manage a swim, but only half as many lengths as I could do before. And after each day I exercised, I would need to have a rest day.

To begin with, we can learn to use physical activity to help us manage the pain, once we have got ourselves sorted out with medication.

Rest and sleep

Even the healthiest human needs sleep. It is one of the four essentials to life, along with air, food and water. Both the amount of sleep and quality of sleep are important to healing and well-being.

For the body to repair itself and recover, rest is essential after exercise and other forms of physical activity. There is not a great deal of point in starting an exercise regime if you are not getting enough rest. Which means getting a good night's sleep and taking a nap during the day if necessary. My mum took a half-hour nap religiously every afternoon. This habit started when she had PMR, over 25 years ago. I was at work and was unable to. Maybe it goes some way to explaining how Mother managed to recover in two years, while it took me four and a half, and how she lived into her 90s. On the other hand, some sleep experts maintain that sleeping during the daytime can interfere with the quality of your sleep at night, so it's very much an issue of personal preference.

Good sleep starts with good "sleep hygiene", which refers to the environment in which we sleep, our routines, and our behaviours around bedtime. This doesn't have to be costly and is in fact surprisingly straightforward. It starts with setting a regular schedule for going to bed to sleep. Bed is for sleeping in, not watching TV, not eating and drinking, not for anything else (except sex, in which case good luck to you). Work out how much sleep you think you need and your preferred waking up time. Then work out what time you need to go to bed. You don't need to have an early night unless you're an early riser. Next, have the best bedding you can afford - make getting into bed a pleasure. Don't have the bedroom too warm. About 18 degrees centigrade is fine. Some people like gentle calming scents such as lavender and geranium to help them into a relaxed state of mind.

Posture when lying down is also important. If we lie on our side, our legs and spine get out of alignment. The weight of the leg on top pushes downwards, compressing the lower part of the body. This distortion then carries through to the rest of our bodies, so we are constantly shifting around trying to find a more comfortable position. A physiotherapist recommended me, a side sleeper, to lie with a pillow between my knees to keep my legs and back aligned, and at times when my back has been playing up, I have found this helpful. It also seems to help reduce the tossing and turning.

For back sleepers, the problem can be due to arching of the lower back. Again, the trusty pillow comes into service, this time underneath the knees. This can make an amazing difference to back and neck comfort in bed.

No amount of pillow talk will make any difference if the mattress has had it. General advice is a mattress, even a good one, only has a life of about seven to ten years. Mattress manufacturers *would* say this, I know. Well, take it from the UK's Sleep Charity[54]. If you are sleeping on an old mattress and have PMR, get yourself sorted out with a new one! This will be your biggest investment in your sleep, but it could also pay dividends in a quicker and more complete recovery. Not to mention the other health benefits of having a good night's sleep. It does not need to be a hard orthopaedic mattress. The most important thing is it should give support to the whole body, all the time. Many older people prefer a slightly softer mattress, and this can be better for you because it allows the body to sink in where it needs to.

I have recently been suffering with insomnia. I believe it was triggered by a period of extreme anxiety about one of our children. One of the lessons of later life is that parenting never stops. There's a lot of truth in the saying "You're only as happy as your unhappiest child". It's lonely and distressing to be wide awake at three in the morning, as the early hours of the morning are when our levels of inflammatory chemicals in the bloodstream such as IL-6 are at their highest. Sleeplessness might be compounded by physical discomfort as well. Sleeping tablets can seem appealing, but doctors are cautious because some can lead to dependence and reduced effectiveness over time.

Researchers have discovered that psychological remedies, in particular, cognitive behavioural therapy (CBT) can be more effective over the long term than pharmaceutical treatments. A core idea is that in cases of chronic sleeplessness, one's brain has learned to associate lying in bed with lying awake, rather than going to sleep. It takes quite a bit of self-discipline to get up in the middle of the night when you think you have been awake for a quarter of an hour. However, I found the programme described in the book I read very effective indeed[55]. I also learned much about sleep patterns and sleep requirements in later life, and since going through the programme (which only took a couple of weeks to put me right), I have stopped worrying about the odd bad night. There is also a wealth of information on the website of the US-based Sleep Foundation[56].

Travel and holidays

There's no reason why you shouldn't enjoy travelling and a good holiday while you have PMR or GCA, though as with any chronic illness, you will need to put some extra thought into planning ahead. I know that quite a few members of the PMRGCAuk online forum on HealthUnlocked are seasoned travellers and have worked it up to a fine art, so I asked them for their suggestions and advice. These quotes are organised into sections: Planning, On the Journey, and While You're There.

Planning

> *"Start your break by booking airport assistance - and you stand a chance of arriving at your destination feeling reasonably human. If it is a long trip to the airport by car - travel the day before and have a night in a hotel."* (PMRpro)

> *"On the subject of travel, it's perhaps worth mentioning that travellers should check with the country they are going to visit that their medicines are not banned or on the controlled list. Who knew that Dubai had an issue with Pregabalin and Diazepam, for example? Also, some countries are quite strict and require a letter from your doctor listing each medicine with amounts prescribed."* (Ancient Aunt)

> *"Think twice about travelling to a part of the world where there's a good chance of you picking up a mosquito-borne virus."* (Christopher)

> *"If you're going somewhere that involves a lot of walking, book for twice as long. We spent a week in Rome doing*

everything most people do in 3 days. It took the pressure off and meant we could take our time." (Broseley)

"If you have adrenal insufficiency, addisonsdisease.org.uk has a wonderful document under the travel page which is a translation into many languages of instructions for a doctor or hospital in another country should you suffer an adrenal crisis there."

"Take special assistance, take any walking aids you may need, take all your meds plus extra, plan a couple of nights to rest from the journey before being more adventurous."

"Make sure you take your emergency steroid cards with you. If possible, take a local language translation as well if going to a non-English-speaking country. Consider getting a bracelet before you go."

To these great ideas I would add:

Do research on your accommodation options and, if you can, book a room in a place that also offers a lounge for guests. If you find you need a rest day, at least then you won't be stuck in one cramped room. Travel light and take only the most comfortable footwear with you.

On the journey

"Take all your medications in your hand luggage and don't let it out of your sight - even Ryanair accept you aren't going to let your hand luggage with medications be checked in for their convenience! Take at least 3 times the amount of pred you think you will need - just in case.

"Book private transport to transfer between the airport and the hotel and back. It saves stress and walking around finding public transport." (PMRpro)

While you're there

"If you can't do something at home without payback - don't assume it'll be fine on holiday!! If you struggle with the stairs at home, you probably won't be walking up the 199 steps to the abbey at Whitby in temperatures in the mid-teens - and you are even less likely to manage 100 steps to an apartment on the cliffs in Greece in temperatures in the low 30s!!"(PMRPro).

"I was diagnosed last Spring and did a not too strenuous walking holiday in Spain in the autumn, on 9mg pred. I had good advice here about being cautious and allowing for rest days, warned my husband we might need to have 'sit on the beach and take public transport' days......and it all went very well. We were walking while our baggage was transferred to the next stop, and I took two lots of prednisolone with me, one to carry, one to leave in my suitcase, just in case either went missing somehow." (Ancient Aunt)

"I find my Garmin really helpful for pacing myself especially the "body battery" feature which shows rest and stress - it's good for reminding you to take a break." (Suzy1959)

"Be realistic about what you can manage and rejoice that we can do it, just a bit differently!"

Suzy has a very positive attitude towards adventurous travel:

"I put off going to Costa Rica for years as I had found long haul flights always resulted in a flare. I bit the bullet and went last year. Flew business class, had an individual itinerary through my travel agent, took private wildlife tours so I didn't slow anyone down and could stop when I had had enough. I did actually cry every day (some anxiety and some

pain). However, it was a wonderful holiday, and I have some great memories."

Vanessa and I have discussed the temptation you might feel to bump up your medication a little as a ruse to ward off symptoms while you are travelling or staying abroad. It's understandable to want some reassurance, but we don't recommend raising your dose. Similarly, although on holiday you might be relaxing and feeling nice, it's not a good idea to reduce either.

Those who do increase their dose might say that it's only for a couple of weeks, but it is part of the pattern of increased dosing for minor stresses that can lead to "stuck" or "yo-yo" dosing, making subsequent tapering more difficult and increasing the risk of cumulative steroid toxicity and adrenal suppression over time.

The rationale for avoiding dose reduction while on holiday is twofold. First, holidays are typically short, and most people understandably wish to minimise the risk of a flare during a long-anticipated break. Second, access to appropriate medical advice or follow-up is often more limited when away from home. That said, this approach would need to be reconsidered in people experiencing significant steroid-related adverse effects, where ongoing dose reduction remains important.

Of course, not everyone has the will or the wherewithal to travel round the world, and it's important to be aware that some people are just too ill with PMR or GCA to even contemplate such things. In response to my request for travel tips, this *cri de coeur* from 'Aging Feminist' arrived:

"I would like to be the voice for people with PMR who have steroid induced muscle myopathy. Go on holiday? What a ridiculous idea...I can only walk about 200 metres and then need recovery time. Use a wheelchair? Sitting in a chair is a tremendous strain on my back muscles. I work full-time (online) lying back on pillows in my bed. Except for medical

appointments and the odd 100-200 metre walk, I haven't left my home for 5 years. I am not alone. Others have complications due to other diseases crowding in."

Yes, Aging Feminist, I hear you. How much we travel, and whether we travel at all, is going to be a matter for careful thought and negotiation with your loved ones. Don't allow anyone to bully you into committing to a trip that you have serious reservations about. They need to understand your abilities and your limitations while you have PMR and GCA. We shouldn't try to cover up all the time.

Nutrition and diet

As PMR and GCA are inflammatory conditions, many people ask whether there are any dietary changes they can make to reduce inflammation in the body. Take this information as a guide only, as there is no established research evidence regarding treatment of PMR and GCA with diets or supplements. I can say this with some confidence, because the international group working on the PMR guidelines carried out an exhaustive literature search and were not able to find any reliable research on the topic.

This is not to say that there is no common wisdom about the role of nutrition in health and recovery from illness and there is generic evidence of the benefit of eating a well-balanced diet, eating enough protein, and eating fresh food, especially vegetables.

Later in this section I report on a very interesting discussion Vanessa and I had with a dietician specialising in helping people living with diabetes and helping the public understand the scientific basis for claims that are made about dietary changes.

As we know, the most common way to treat PMR and GCA is taking steroids. During the acute stage, medication is indispensable. However, after the acute stage, some people would like to help themselves towards recovery through diet and nutrition, hoping that this will enable them to reduce their steroid intake or eliminate it altogether. Before you plan to do so, I strongly advise that you mention this to your GP or rheumatologist to make sure you're not overlooking any particular risks (though, as Vanessa points out to me, they are not trained to discuss all diet-related issues!). There is a lot of discussion online among patient groups in which individuals claim, for example, that cutting out 'nightshades' such as tomatoes has done wonders for their inflammation levels. Take all such claims with the legendary pinch of salt.

The British Heart Foundation website has some helpful advice about claims that certain foods help to reduce inflammation. While recognising that, for example, blueberries, olive oil, turmeric and oily fish might have anti-inflammatory properties, they point out that any studies suggesting this have been carried out in labs using concentrated extracts from these foods, so it's unclear whether these foods would have any effects in the human body as part of a wider diet.

Where studies have been done on the food intake of whole populations, we can see the strongest evidence of food effects by comparing the general diet with the incidence of certain diseases in that population. This is where the evidence in favour of the so-called Mediterranean diet comes from, where a high intake of fresh fruit and vegetables, quality unsaturated oils and fresh fish seems to have an impact on overall prevalence of heart disease in the population. Any apparent anti-inflammatory effects (note that heart disease may be linked to inflammation) seem to come from a range of foods working together.

Diet, not nutrients

This part of the chapter follows a familiar structure of looking at different types of nutrients and discussing how they affect our health. However, it's worth mentioning that in recent years, a different approach has become popular among nutrition experts in the US and UK, focusing on diet as a whole rather than individual components. People don't eat nutrients - they eat food. What's more, they eat food in the context of a more general diet and approach to eating. Eating healthily once a day isn't going to help an awful lot if the rest of the time, we are grabbing fatty, ultra-processed snacks.

The Dietary Approach to Stopping Hypertension eating plan (DASH), aimed at helping reduce high blood pressure, has become popularised in the US and UK, because it provides this more holistic approach[57] It emphasises a balanced pattern of eating, rich in fruit, vegetables, whole grains, and low-fat dairy, rather than focusing on individual "superfoods." A Cambridge University epidemiology unit has published findings to support the adoption of the DASH eating plan, ideally across the public as a whole, but has also identified certain barriers to adopting it wholesale. Two of these, I think, are particularly relevant to older people with PMR and GCA. They have found that people living on their own are less likely to be eating healthily than people who are married or in relationships. Many of us in later life find ourselves alone and may not put as much effort into preparing and eating the right kinds of food as when we had our partner to think about too. In fact, half of the people over 75 in the UK are living alone. The second is that evidence shows a lack of social ties among older people is associated, particularly among men, with eating a smaller variety of fruit and vegetables.

Protein

Don't think that because you are getting older, and not growing or reproducing any more, you don't need protein. We all need a certain amount of protein to help repair damaged cells and maintain optimum working of the various systems in our bodies. Some nutritionists suggest processed red meats can increase inflammation in the body.

Calcium

In patient information, such as the ArthritisUK leaflets[58], emphasis is placed on the risk of developing osteoporosis when you are on steroids. You should eat calcium-rich foods, and if not, take a calcium supplement. The Mayo Clinic, for instance, recommends incorporating whole grains, sufficient calcium and vitamin D, as well as low-fat meat. This could help to mitigate risk of thinning bones, high blood pressure and diabetes. Many also recommend oily fish, like sardines, herring, trout and wild salmon. All this adds up to a low inflammatory diet.

According to the British Dietetic Association, an ideal calcium intake for adults is 700mg-1000mg daily. To assess the calcium you are taking in, use the table below. Each point equates to 50mg of calcium, so aim for at least 14 points a day:

Points	Calcium sources
5	One pot plain or fruit yoghurt, or one third pint milk or 2oz (50g or half a tin) sardines in tomato sauce, or 2oz (50g) tofu
4	One ounce (25g) Cheddar cheese, or a large serving leafy green veg or one third pint calcium enriched soya milk.
3	One tablespoon Parmesan cheese, or 2oz (50g) tinned pilchards in tomato sauce, or one scoop of dairy ice cream, or 3 dried figs, or 2 slices white or wholemeal bread, or a small pot of calcium-enriched soya yoghurt.
2	One pot fromage frais, or half a small tin of salmon, or 4oz (small tub) cottage cheese, or small bar milk chocolate, or half a large tin of kidney beans.
1	One third pint soya milk, or 3 heaped tsp Horlicks, or one small tin baked beans, or 9 Brazil nuts or 8 dried apricot halves, or 5 oz (125g) boiled cabbage.

Table 3: Dietary sources of Calcium: the points system

Vitamin D

Adequate vitamin D is also important to maintain bone strength. We need vitamin D to help us to extract the calcium from our food. Unfortunately, low or suboptimal vitamin D levels are common in the UK especially in the winter. The housebound are particularly vulnerable because their bodies are not making vitamin D in response to sunlight. Dietary sources include oily fish, liver, egg yolks, fortified juices and some breakfast cereals, and vitamin D enriched milk, but unless you love oily fish and have it daily, you are likely to fall short, especially in the UK winter. If you are on steroids, you should also be taking a vitamin D supplement, but even when you come off the steroids, continue keeping the supplement up, especially if you are over 70 or have dark skin. These are not generally available on prescription, but you can buy a four-month supply for about £10.

Magnesium

Recent research points to the role magnesium plays in regulating the immune response and thus the levels of inflammation in the body[59]. Low intake of magnesium is associated (not necessarily causally linked) with chronic conditions such as Type 2 diabetes, hypertension and cardiovascular disease, particularly in older and overweight people. Low levels of magnesium have been associated with higher CRP readings in humans. However, the way magnesium operates on inflammation in the case of chronic musculoskeletal conditions is poorly understood, because the necessary studies haven't been done.

Food sources of magnesium include dark leafy greens, like spinach and kale, peas and beans, soy products, whole grains and low-fat dairy. Fish is another good source. A lot of magnesium in food is lost during production processes such as refining white flour, and the body generally will only absorb about 40% of the magnesium we consume. For me, the message is not to invest in magnesium supplements, but to make sure we eat plenty of the right foods and avoid ultra-processed food as much as possible.

Vanessa says: on magnesium

Whilst magnesium has roles in immune function and is associated with inflammatory markers, there is no good clinical evidence that increasing magnesium intake improves outcomes in inflammatory rheumatic diseases such as PMR or GCA. There is limited and mixed evidence for benefit in conditions like insomnia (poor sleep), migraine and fibromyalgia, but effects are modest, inconsistent and not disease-modifying. Optimising dietary intake with Kate's advice is reasonable and will probably have wider health benefits, but magnesium supplements are generally not recommended for people with GCA or PMR unless deficiency is present.

---- x ----

Fruit and veg

We have become very used to the litany from health professionals that we need to increase our intake of fresh fruits and vegetables – the famous "five a day". Just about any vegetables are really good for us, and the best thing we can do is ensure a good balance between roots, such as swedes, turnips and carrots; leaves, such as cabbage and chard; stems such as celery and asparagus; seeds, such as peas and beans; and fruits, such as tomatoes and peppers.

Vegetables are of course bursting with vitamins and minerals, as well as fibre, and some are a source of protein too. Keep fresh vegetables in the fridge to improve keeping and delay loss of nutrients. Remember too that frozen vegetables are just as nutritious as fresh. It is common knowledge that some of the vitamin content of vegetables is lost in the cooking water. Vitamin C, being water-soluble, is the most vulnerable of the vitamins from this point of view. Others, such as the fat-soluble Vitamins E and K, are not so likely to be lost. When boiling vegetables, use as little water as you can get away with. Try steaming or microwaving them instead. Microwaving works by causing water molecules in the food to oscillate and generate heat. Because the cooking times are shorter, any increased heat damage is balanced out by the quicker cooking. Contrary to popular opinion, cooking vegetables thoroughly won't necessarily reduce their nutritional value when you eat them[60]. You might reduce the nutritional content to some extent, but when a vegetable is properly cooked, your digestive system will be more able to extract all the goodness from it. So, if you have a delicate digestion and prefer your vegetables cooked rather than raw, do not worry about it.

It does seem that for us, whole fruits and vegetables are better than fruit juice. This is because a glass of juice holds the sugars of the fruit in concentration, and fruit sugar, or fructose, is absorbed very quickly by the body. Better to eat the orange segments, because of the fibre content.

Supplements and special foods

Going back to the question of anti-inflammatory foods, many people experiment with certain foods and substances claimed to reduce inflammation in the body. For example, curcumin, which is a substance in the spice turmeric, has been observed in experimental conditions to have an effect on the C-reactive protein signals inflammation in blood tests. However, nobody really knows how much curcumin you should eat in a 'normal diet' to make a difference, or quite what the mechanism is reducing the CRP[61].

Other foods, such as members of the solanum, or nightshade, family, are thought by some people to make inflammation worse. These foods are peppers (capsicums), aubergines, tomatoes and potatoes. Unfortunately, these last two are important ingredients in the diet of many older British people! I have done some research into this and, to be honest, I have not been able to find a single piece of convincing published peer-reviewed research supporting the idea that these vegetables increase inflammation in the body. Certain websites claim this scientific research exists while not telling us what it is. Don't trust them.

I followed one link on such a website back to another site that presented a published paper – from 1993. This reported second-hand information about inflammation observed in livestock after they had been eating the stems and leaves of plants from the solanum (nightshade) family. Thankfully, our diets are a bit more varied than the diet of the average cow. What is more, the concentration of the alkaloid substance that is the source of this concern is much lower in the fruits and roots of these plants than in the stems and leaves. This is because it is part of the plant's defence system, giving leaves and stems a bitter taste to repel the bugs. I am not about to start eating tomato leaves, so I'm not going to worry about this, and I will carry on enjoying tomatoes and even the odd aubergine. These foods are full of nutritious value, including antioxidants associated with supporting bone health and other aspects of our body's amazing systems.

Food sensitivities

This is not to say, of course, there aren't certain people with an inbuilt sensitivity to certain foods, foods that literally disagree with them. So, if you have a sensitive tummy, and if you can afford it, it might be worth your while trying to find out which foods might make you feel worse, and which might make you feel better. The way to do this is to cut out certain food groups (dairy, nightshades, wheat, for example) from your diet for three to four weeks. This will give your system time to adjust, although this approach is not strongly evidence-based for inflammatory conditions. Keep a diary of your symptoms during this time. Then introduce the foods again, one at a time, for one day at a time. Then monitor for two days. So, for example, you might introduce bread on Tuesday and monitor yourself on Wednesday and Thursday for reactions. Then on Friday, try a different food. This way of identifying what you may be intolerant to is exhaustive, and you need to plan and be very organized and stick to it.

Vanessa reminds me that elimination diets are used in specific conditions (mainly irritable bowel syndrome and allergy) but are not well supported for inflammatory rheumatic disease. However, it might be fun, and it could give you really valuable information about your personal dietary dos and don'ts.[62] As for me, I simply wouldn't have the self-discipline to see it through.

I wrote in the last edition about how I took pure aloe juice every day while trying to get off steroids. I convinced myself if it wasn't doing any good, at least it wasn't doing any harm. I told myself a story about healing my "leaky gut". But I no longer believe we need special foods for our gut. To be honest, while you're recovering from PMR or GCA I would recommend just eating a varied diet with as much fresh quality food, particularly leafy greens, as you can afford and be kind to yourself.

A dietician's take on inflammation

During our research for this book, Vanessa and I had a very interesting meeting with Duane Miller, who is a Senior Specialist Dietitian in the south of England.

Duane confirmed our suspicion that, for most people, there isn't a simple fix when it comes to diet and inflammatory illnesses. Many people make claims for the role of antioxidants in the diet, but Duane says, while they work to some extent 'in the test tube' the effects of foods and specific substances on the actual human body is much more complex. Turmeric in particular sounds very promising, but the fact is, it's very difficult for the body to absorb it, and one would have to eat an awful lot of it for it to make any difference to someone with an inflammatory illness like PMR or GCA. Small amounts, he says, may have a minor effect, but not a medicinal effect. That is to say, while eating foods richly seasoned with turmeric may help a bit, and certainly not do you any harm, they will be no substitute for your prescribed medication.

We talked about the evidence of some people with Rheumatoid Arthritis experiencing an improvement in their symptoms by following the so-called Mediterranean Diet. So far so good. But Duane believes the key here is not so much magic ingredients such as tomatoes or olive oil or fancy seasonings, but the fact the Med diet is rich in vegetables, and simple fresh ingredients in season. As long as it's fresh, containing lots of seasonal vegetables, it could be any cuisine - Chinese, French, even British. Carrots and cabbage can be just as good for you as olives and aubergines! Duane's question to you is "What do you enjoy? What can you maintain as a pattern of cooking and eating for life?" I'd also add – "what is most affordable and local?"

Breakfast

Breakfast is a really important meal. Duane's advice is to go for lots of fibre and protein in the morning rather than a whole lot of carbohydrates. If you have a high carb breakfast, such as packaged cereal, or toast and marmalade, you may bring on blood sugar spikes because you take your steroids in the morning.

A few years ago, my husband was struggling with Long Covid, and I was feeling I really needed to get to grips with my Type 2 diabetes. I found a source of information online that included occasional webinars. One of these was with an American gastroenterologist. She said, while common wisdom used to be that fibre helped our bowels to be regular by keeping digested food moving through our intestines, it has been established that the gut flora, the bacteria so crucial to our general health, actually feed on dietary fibre. She recommended starting the day by "priming" your gut with a green smoothie, a mix of vegetables like celery, green leaves and cucumber, with fruit like banana and apple. Add a handful of porridge oats, a slosh of dairy or non-dairy milk, a dollop of yoghurt and some water, and blitz the lot in the centrifugal blender. She said, "You don't have to like it, you just have to drink it." But we started and we've found it surprisingly pleasant.

We can't claim this habit has solved all our health issues, but we certainly don't get hungry in the morning, and our gut health is as good as it has ever been, if not better. So, I'm all for the idea of fibre in the morning. (At this point Vanessa will want to make a disclaimer about not being able to verify this with established evidence, but in this case I'm comfortable with that!). In fact, recent research funded by ArthritisUK, carried out by a team based at University College London[63], has established that imbalances and shortages in gut flora, the *gut microbiome* as it's known, can contribute to the development and severity of rheumatoid arthritis. So why would it not also be relevant to other chronic inflammatory illnesses?

If you read posts on PMR and GCA groups on Facebook, you'll see there's a common feeling among people who've lived with PMR and/or GCA for a long time, that super-low carbohydrate diets are helpful, to mitigate weight gain and even counteract inflammation. Duane says in the nutritionist world there are "low-carb communities", that is, people who are very much in favour of restricting carbohydrate intake as much as possible. They believe carbohydrates get "oxidised" on being consumed by the body, and this is part of the inflammatory process. But according to Duane, there isn't really any firm evidence that an extreme low carb diet is anti-inflammatory. This idea is more based on a theoretical perspective than on real-life evidence. But it can be very empowering and psychologically helpful for some individuals who want to feel they have found their own path towards recovery. There is absolutely nothing wrong with that.

There is also quite a lot of controversy about fats. Some people are advocates of fish oils. According to Duane, the results of fish oil studies are not conclusive, but there is very limited evidence of any harm. I take from this, if you want to take a fish oil supplement, go ahead, but there's no guarantee it will make any difference to your overall health, still less your PMR or GCA. As far as seed oils are concerned, there are some claims they can contribute to inflammation, but again, the evidence is very weak. If you remove ultra-processed food from your diet (food items containing ingredients you wouldn't find in your own storage cupboard), you will probably be reducing your intake of saturated fats, which have been linked to high cholesterol and vascular damage. On the other hand, if you eat meat and butter occasionally, there probably won't be a major threat from the saturated fat in those. Again, the message is to eat fresh, natural and simple.

Be healthily sceptical about any diet heralded as the answer to inflammation. There's no magic bullet. There is some evidence according to Duane that the practice of intermittent fasting might be of some benefit, but again, the evidence on human physiology is pretty weak. Scrolling through different types of diets might be a distraction, but it's not going to be the answer.

Vanessa (from her clinical practice) and I (from experience) are very conscious that you can spend a long time with the munchies when you are on steroids. In other words, you're hungry practically all the time. We asked Duane if he has any tips for managing hunger. He referred back to the importance of breakfast. It's your first conscious eating decision of the day, and so if you choose your breakfast meal wisely, it can set the pattern for the rest of the day. Protein and fibre can help fill you up. For example, egg and beans, or egg and wholemeal toast, can keep you going well into the day. Duane says it helps to eat mindfully, thinking of what you are doing and eating in that moment, slowing down to appreciate the food and the act of eating. If you're eating too quickly, he says, you are not giving your body a chance to respond to being fed.

Another tip for staving off hunger pangs later in the day is to carry on with the protein and fibre pattern, for example with bean soups, or vegetable and lentil soups (Duane is a big fan of soups, as am I, especially if they're homemade). Ask yourself whether you are really hungry or could you just actually be thirsty. Try having a drink and a small healthy snack and check out whether your hunger pangs are still there. If you can build some distraction by socialising into your daily routine, so much the better.

Treats

The idea of socialising brought our conversation round to the topic of cake. Cake is everywhere in British culture: it seems to be a national obsession. And for older retired people who brighten their lives with visits to cafes, either alone, with a partner, or to meet friends, cake is the first thing you see when you walk along the counter to order your cappuccino. When we were children in the fifties and sixties, cake was still a luxury, a treat. There might be a Swiss-roll on payday, and a homemade fruit cake on Sunday. But today, eating cake seems to have acquired a special status in our lives. Refusing a piece of cake can almost feel as though we are being party-poopers, or quietly criticising the people who are tucking into huge wedges of salted caramel double chocolate sponge. And why would you not want to give yourself a treat when you're putting up with PMR or GCA?

Well, Duane's answer to this is we can't expect to change our eating environment to how it was in Crete in the 1950s. Fair enough Duane. Instead, he suggests taking control. Even if the Government gets its act together to tax ultra-processed food, the "eating environment", he says, will still leave a lot to be desired. So, what would taking control look like?

Give yourself permission to eat a safe amount of treat foods like cake or chocolate. In a social situation, why not accept the cake and just eat half of it? Better still, buy one slice to share between two - a way of sharing the love. Don't be crippled by guilt. Giving yourself permission can in fact be empowering and make you feel more in control.

Plan your route through the supermarket to get to the things you actually want to buy while avoiding the things you don't. Supermarkets are masters at end-of-aisle offers and the treats they put at eye-level to tempt you. Think of the money you'll save by not falling for them. Of course, if you go supermarket shopping with a partner, you'll need to enlist their support for this. Sociologists have noted that children who were born during, or soon after, the era of rationing (I, in my seventies, am one of them) grew up in a culture of not wasting anything, of eating everything on your plate whether it was palatable or not. Then, a little later after the end of the war, as life became more affluent, a culture of treating yourself or treating the kids came in (like getting an ice-cream from the Mr Whippy van). Sugar became a metaphor for love. But there are other ways of being nice to ourselves. We need to recognise what they are for us and value them as much as foodie treats.

Weight gain

We came to the bugbear of anyone who has put on what feels like a ton of weight since starting steroid medication. How do you lose weight? Some people swear by shake-based diets, using commercially bought mixes that fill you up and fill your basic nutritional needs. By now you won't be surprised that Duane isn't a big fan of these either. However, they can be a help temporarily if people are struggling to lose weight.

Similarly, the GLP1 weight loss drugs are causing a stir and quite a lot of PMR and GCA sufferers online are reporting using these and getting results. That is, the result they are looking for is losing the excess weight they have put on since starting steroids. And the battle of fighting the steroid hunger can last a year or more while you are tapering to more of a maintenance level. These drugs can be effective in the short term, but we need to rethink our relationship with food, and its place in our lives, our wellbeing and our self-esteem, otherwise after the drugs, the problems will just come back.

An effect of the weight loss drugs less often talked about is that they are hitting bone health and muscle mass, because of the speed of the weight loss affecting tissue formation and renewal. If you have PMR or GCA and you have the weight loss jabs, they are disrupting your natural process at the same time the steroids are hitting at your bones and muscles as well. So do think carefully about optimising your nutrition, exercise, and bone protection medication as needed, and discuss with your doctor before going onto drugs like Mounjaro.

Vanessa thinks GLP1 drugs are potentially an exciting area in inflammatory diseases. At the moment, there are no clinical trials supporting their use for PMR or GCA. However, early research suggests they may have modest effects on inflammation, so it's possible that in the future they could be explored as an add-on therapy, especially for patients with metabolic issues like diabetes or excess weight, but for now, their use for PMR or GCA remains purely experimental.

We have a whole chapter on exercise and activity in this book, but let's just make a connection right here, because what we eat and how we use and move our bodies is fundamental to our overall health and wellbeing as we age, whether or not we have a chronic condition like PMR or GCA. Think about body shape and size, and your overall condition, not so much focused on how you look but about how well you are functioning. Focus on eating and exercise to maintain your bone density, keeping your muscle mass as much as possible, and keeping mobile, because the chances are you will get through the PMR and GCA and you'll want to be in the best shape possible going forward. Store up the benefit for the future. You won't be sorry.

Finally, on a personal note, allow me to share with you what I believe about eating when you have a chronic health condition. I am no nutritional expert, but I have read a lot, listened a lot, and thought a lot about it. And eaten a lot too! I think it basically boils down to a few principles:

1. Make sure you eat enough. Eat at least three times a day, preferably four, including a little snack before bedtime to help you through the night. Eat fresh as often as possible and avoid ultra-processed foods. Fresh doesn't necessarily mean raw though. Older people may absorb more nutrients from cooked food.
2. Keep your food varied. A little bit of everything and everything in moderation.
3. Don't beat yourself up about putting on some weight while you are taking steroids. There may be very little you can do about it for now. Speak with your doctor about your weight concerns and concentrate on getting your dosage right for you, rather than fretting about diet. I put on seven kilos but lost them during the year after coming off steroids without having to diet.
4. When you go out for a restaurant meal, go for the starter and the main but pass on the dessert. Restaurants make big profits on puddings full of fat and sugar, bought in, and frankly, not very nice. Be kind to yourself and refuse them. After a while, you won't miss them and if you do have a portion of pavlova, it will make you feel nauseous. Don't be afraid to ask if you can share a starter if the portions coming out of the kitchen look big. You can even have two starters instead of one plus a main.
5. When facing something very fatty, however delicious it looks, picture in your mind the fat in that dish as a lump of lard sitting in the middle of your plate. Disgusting! Will you eat it? No, of course you won't!
6. No diets while you have a chronic illness. No fasting, no 5:2 diet, no anything. Just good simple food and enough of

it. Crash dieting will put your body under stress and just upset your immune system even more.

GCA and aneurysm - should I be worried?

We've spoken about GCA being a vasculitis, and the large vessels being involved. You may have read on social media or the forum that if you have, or have had, GCA, your risk of getting an aneurysm is higher than the rest of the population. This is not untrue, and thinking about aneurysm is scary, but it's important to keep this in perspective and not worry yourself too much about it. Vanessa has written a note to help us understand.

Vanessa says: on aortic aneurysm

In some people with GCA, inflammation affects the wall of the thoracic aorta (the part passing through the chest). Over time, this inflammation, or damage left behind by past inflammation, can weaken the artery wall and cause it to widen. This widening is called an aneurysm.

Overall, about 10 to 15 out of every 100 people with GCA will develop an aortic aneurysm at some point[64,65]. However, routine screening of all patients with GCA is not recommended in most countries. This is because most people never develop an aneurysm, and many aneurysms that do occur remain small, stable, and never cause harm. Detecting these can lead to repeated scans and anxiety without clear benefit. Even when larger aneurysms are found, treatment involves major surgery, which carries significant risk, especially in older people or those with other medical conditions: in many cases, the risks outweigh the benefits.

It is also important to keep this risk in perspective. People are of course most worried about a rupture of an aneurysm, because it's almost always fatal. But most people with GCA do not die from aneurysm rupture. Cardiovascular disease, such as heart attack or stroke, accounts for around 40–50 out of every 100 deaths. Infection and cancer each account for roughly 10–20 out of 100 deaths. Aortic complications account for a much smaller proportion, probably around 1–2 in every 100 deaths, with rupture itself even rarer.

Screening with imaging like CT or MRI may be appropriate for selected higher-risk patients. These include those with evidence of aortic inflammation on imaging, those with widespread or persistent disease, younger patients at diagnosis, and those with additional risk factors such as smoking, high blood pressure, or male sex.

Aneurysms typically develop slowly, often many years after diagnosis, most commonly around 7 to 10 years. There is no universally agreed screening schedule, and decisions are usually individualised.

People with PMR on its own do not seem to have a much higher risk of developing an aortic aneurysm than the general population[63]. If your GCA was limited to the arteries in the head, and responded well to treatment, your risk is likely low. If large vessels were involved, your risk is higher, and this is worth discussing with your doctor.

Finally, reducing overall cardiovascular risk is important for everyone with GCA or PMR. This includes controlling inflammation, managing blood pressure and cholesterol, looking out for diabetes and avoiding smoking.

---- x ----

NHS Emergency Steroid Card

Get yourself kitted out with an NHS Steroid Emergency card if you are in the UK. These cards were introduced by the NHS in 2020 to safeguard people who might suffer from an adrenal insufficiency emergency should their daily steroid dose be suddenly stopped, for example if they are admitted to hospital after a fall.

Building your personal support system

We have a responsibility to educate people around us about PMR and GCA because they are still so little-known, even in the medical world. We're an ageing population and more people will be getting PMR and GCA, and everyone needs to know the symptoms of GCA like they need to know the symptoms of heart attack or stroke. There isn't going to be a revolution in public funding to give the health service every penny it needs to look after everyone. We need to become more independent and more resourceful about our own health, and get our heads round science, learning how to distinguish good from bad science, reliable from cranky information.

After PMR and GCA

I realised, if I live as long as my parents, into my 90s (I hope), I will need to look after myself pretty vigorously in order to keep as fit and mobile as I can into old age. I had to face the fact that, with my stressful lifestyle, a high-powered job in a toxic organisation, a commute 95 miles and back, I wasn't doing any good by my immune system. I was almost addicted to stress in my life. It was hard, and took a long time, to learn how to live without the constant buzz from job stress and allow some space into my life to grow spiritually, rather than putting my energies into achieving in my career and earning money.

Even after I took my pension and gave up commuting to my academic job in Oxford, I transferred my energies to PMRGCAuk and dedicated another six years to nurturing the charity. Thank goodness I realised the changes I was making in my diet and other habits would have to be permanent, for life.

I need sleep. Going without sleep makes me crazy and ill. I need exercise, even if I cannot run half-marathons anymore. Exercise means thinking not only about a brisk walk now and again but systematically planning for regular activities that have different benefits to the body. Swimming for suppleness, dancing for balance, Pilates for muscle strength (I have slipped on this one), walking for bone strength, swimming for cardiovascular and suppleness. I need to keep my intake of sugar down and work hard on controlling diabetes with a minimum of medication. I need to be in touch with nature, and go to the allotment regularly, even if I just sit in the shed and watch the rhubarb grow.

What if it doesn't go away?

It would be great to be like an internet influencer and love bomb you with assurances that PMR and GCA are just temporary conditions and everyone will get better if you take the medicine and eat the right stuff and do the right things. I have to confront the uncomfortable fact that, for some people, a residual form of PMR and/or GCA lingers, perhaps for the rest of their lives. This recognition has come about because the internet, and PMRGCAuk helped by the internet, have brought PMR and GCA sufferers together in a way unimaginable even twenty years ago. The HealthUnlocked forum has created a community of thousands of people who in the past could never have hoped to meet anyone else with PMR or GCA. The in-person and online support groups provide opportunities for individuals to share their experience and learn from each other. And it now cannot be ignored that there are those, perhaps 20% of people, for whom PMR or GCA becomes a lifelong companion. Here is A, who has been on the forum for ten years, sharing her experience:

> *"I'm into year 10 with this bloody condition; two years undiagnosed, then steroids from 2015 onwards.......*
>
> *"There are two main things I've come to understand and I think they're underestimated. A majority will respond as expected and the condition will go into complete remission within 2,3,4 years. But it's almost as if there's a slightly*

different condition where for a significant minority, maybe 20% plus, it doesn't go away. I'm in the latter group but it took me years to realise. This group seems to plateau. Steroids become less effective, there's yoyo-ing, other meds may be offered or tried. I talked about methotrexate with GP and we agreed it's not a guaranteed solution and no ride in the park. I'm staying with what I have and self-managing. Further rheumatology referral seems a waste of time.

"And that brings me to the other thing; acceptance and mental health. There's a recent paper showing the effect of chronic pain is poorly understood and the effect on the individual is unclear. I'm a positive person. I've enjoyed good health and life, and I try to be equable.

"That said, there are days when getting through is a real struggle. I've had to learn to focus on small pleasures and shut out the negatives and it's not easy. I'm resolute but it's come close to breaking me. It's a condition that requires mental strength and accepting that there's no magic wand to make it go away is part of the 'treatment'."

I'm really grateful to A, for her openness and honesty in this account of her experience.

Find distraction

Don't dwell too much on what is happening in your body. Spending hours of the day monitoring yourself, your mobility, your fatigue level, your pain, can lower your mood. It would be surprising if it didn't. Avoid thinking of yourself as an invalid. Polymyalgia rheumatica or giant cell arteritis are what you have, they are not what you are. You cannot walk away from your condition, but you can stop it defining you. There is still so much to live for, even if you have less energy than you used to have. Don't get into a downward spiral - depression lurks at the bottom. Find what helps you to shift attention away from your body's inward feelings and outwards into the world. It could be learning a new language, going to an Aquacise class at the baths, pottering around in the garden, helping children learn to read, baking bread. Such activities can take up just one or two hours, and will be tiring, but will give you a sense of achievement and satisfaction.

This chapter has covered a host of topic areas all connected with your general well-being on the road to recovery. If there is one single message that running through everything it will be this - "Be as well as you can be." This might mean making quite a big change in your life, or just small tweaks to shift things a little. Everyone is different. Don't compare yourself with others. I've included my own experiences here, not to be some kind of role model, but for you to notice those differences. Compare it with A's story too and recognise the part luck plays in all this. Don't set yourself unreachable goals. Take life a day at a time and a step at a time. Cherish yourself.

7 Exercise and activity

Contributed by Dr. Anne O'Brien.

Neither I nor Vanessa felt properly qualified to give exercise advice to you, who might have other health issues besides your PMR or GCA. So, we asked senior academic physiotherapist Professor Anne O'Brien of Keele University for her ideas on this. Anne generously offered to write a chapter, based on her years of experience researching the benefits of physiotherapy for people with PMR.

Here, Anne focuses on PMR, but exercise is also really important for those with GCA. We have already discussed that steroids weaken your muscles, thin your bones, and reduce your fitness over time. Regular exercise helps counteract these effects by keeping your muscles strong, supporting bone health, and maintaining your balance and stamina.

From here on, the words are Anne's, and the illustrations are by Dr Matthew Baxter, of the University of Leeds.

Introduction

Are you feeling tempted to skip this chapter, wondering how on earth exercise and activity could possibly help when you're already in pain and feel exhausted? If so, hold on and just read a bit further.

Everyone's journey is different with PMR or GCA, but for all of us, keeping moving usually has multiple benefits as we get older. By keeping as fit and mobile as possible, we can live our best lives while recovering from PMR and GCA. We can keep active, and still physically do as many as possible of the things we want to do.

How can exercising help me?

The PMR secret you may not have heard is that exercise and activity, if done the correct way, can ease aches and pains, reduce feelings of stiffness and even combat the tiredness you may be experiencing. Although almost no research has yet been undertaken about how movement specifically impacts people living with PMR, a lot of research has been done in other similar conditions. Rheumatoid arthritis is an example where there is quite a lot of evidence about how to exercise safely. So, the contents of this chapter are informed by this research.

I should declare at this point I am a UK physiotherapist and academic having completed a doctorate exploring the role of UK physiotherapists working with people living with PMR[66,67]. This freely downloadable booklet gives you top tips and suggestions about how to keep active, do exercises and promotes the importance and value of keeping moving. So, I am really committed to helping people with PMR keep moving and enabling you to keep as active as possible.

In this chapter, we will elaborate on five areas:

a. Some of the known benefits of physical activity and exercise for all older adults.
b. How having PMR impacts movement and activities of daily life.
c. Listening to our bodies when living with PMR, taking back some control and pacing our activities.
d. Suggesting a few safe and relevant exercises to try to keep supple, keep strong and even get fitter.
e. Top tips to help you get moving with PMR.

Benefits of physical activity and exercise for all older adults

We are always being told we should be moving more, especially as these days our lifestyles are more sedentary than ever before. You probably already know there is a lot of consistent international evidence, including from the World Health Organisation strongly promoting "active and healthy ageing." Many sources warn us about the dangers of inactivity and to counter this, strongly recommend adults do at least 150 minutes of moderate intensity exercise every week to help reduce the risk of serious health issues in older age, including various cancers, cardiovascular conditions, high blood pressure, and Type 2 diabetes.

There is a lot of research summarising the many physical, as well as mental health benefits of older people exercising[68]. And many specialist groups and charities supporting older people[69], and those with arthritic conditions, promote physical activity[70].

In PMR, international clinical guidelines provide specific guidance[3]. However, we also know from other research that keeping active in older age improves our overall quality of life and reduces our risks of becoming disabled in later life[71], so there are lots of good reasons to keep moving (see Table 1), even if it may feel odd and uncomfortable at the start.

Exercise v physical activity

Many of us use the terms exercise and physical activity a lot in daily life, and probably interchangeably, but for the purpose of this chapter, I use them in a specific way, using Caspersen *et al*'s[72] definitions from 1985. Let me explain.

Exercise is planning, structured and repetitive; it may be tailored to an individual and is purposefully designed to achieve something specific. Examples could be exercises to address a weak hand grip or to increase shoulder range of movement or directed to improve overall fitness levels.

Exercise is therefore different from physical activity, which is any bodily movement resulting in energy expenditure. Physical activity is much more generic and incorporates everyday movement activities; like walking around the shops, climbing stairs, doing housework or gardening. So physical activity is not necessarily planned nor specifically trying to achieve something in the body[73]. In the context of living with PMR, and from my own research, I am confident both exercise and physical activity can have a place and will have long term benefits for the body.

Exercising with PMR

You may be thinking, well that's all very well, but, as someone living with PMR, my muscles already ache and my body is stiff much of the time, so exercising is not that easy. On top of that I feel so tired. And of course, you have a good point. Fatigue is increasingly recognised as a real challenge when living with PMR[74]. But people living with other inflammatory musculoskeletal conditions say the same thing. And studies of people living with those conditions consistently demonstrate there can be improvements in pain and fatigue if we keep moving[75].

Research I have done with UK physiotherapists has suggested exercise plays a major part in physiotherapy/physical therapy management of PMR. Of the 1,032 physiotherapists surveyed, 80% thought that people living with PMR benefit from physiotherapy. I should be clear here though. I am not suggesting that everyone with PMR should be referred to physiotherapy. I am saying all movement, be it exercise or just general physical activity in daily life, is likely to help you manage your PMR better, both in the short and the long term.

Known benefit	Examples and relevance in PMR
Improve everyday mobility	Being able to keep shoulders moving freely to dress yourself/ comb your hair
Improve mental health	Keep a positive outlook on life and prepare for recovering from PMR
Improve muscle strength	Keep being able to climb stairs and get on and off the toilet without needing help
Keep independent in activities of daily life	Not needing help with dressing/ washing, turning over in bed or walking
Reduce risk of cardiovascular conditions	Less likelihood of having a heart attack or stroke
Reduce pain, stiffness	Reduce many of the symptoms of PMR
Reduce fatigue and improve sleep	Get some energy back to help you be more active
Reduce risk of becoming frail and falling	By keeping strong and avoiding falls, you may avoid broken bones

Table 4 - Benefits of exercising as an older person, World Health Org.

You are not alone. There are people who may be able to help and give you advice. "Exercise on prescription" is one great UK scheme where you can get individualised advice and an exercise programme to suit your needs and goals. You can ask your family doctor to refer you to get an assessment. But other alternatives exist, including, for example, the "Silver Sneakers" programme in the United States, so it's worth finding out what is out there in your locality.

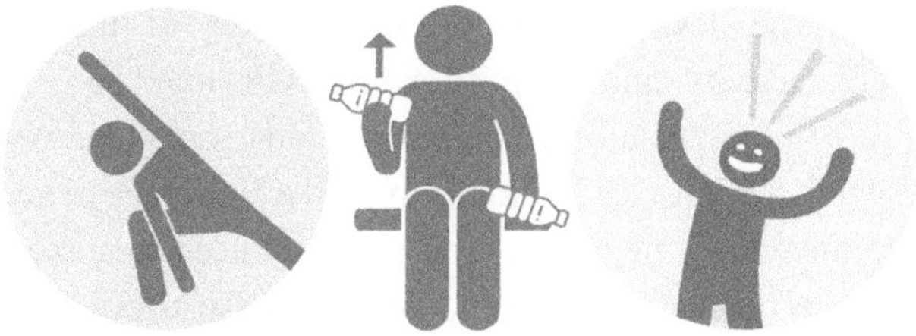

Figure 4: Keep active, strong and mentally positive with PMR and GCA

Little changes can make a big difference

It can all feel a bit overwhelming, but take heart, simple little changes can make a big difference. Keeping it simple is part of the trick to managing this and taking control of your PMR. Here are some examples:

- Make sure to get some fresh air every day. This could be just consciously taking a gentle 10-minute walk down the road or walking the dog a few minutes longer than usual.

- Try to improve your posture by standing tall. Pulling your shoulders back and tummy in, even when sitting in a chair, can help.

- Climb stairs whenever you can, rather than taking a lift.

Remember all these changes make a difference over time.

Starting a new exercise regime can sound expensive and time consuming, but it doesn't have to involve any cost or wearing any Lycra! You really don't need to buy fancy weights or join a gym. Simple everyday changes at home in your daily life will make a real difference.

Activity you enjoy

If you enjoy yoga or Pilates or golf, whatever, go and do it, but take it gently. The PMRGCAuk self-help guide to maintaining movement, activity and exercise with PMR may be a useful reference point, especially if you are planning something new for you. Expect your muscles and joints to need a bit of time to get used to being moved in a new way. And you may need to make a few modifications compared with someone who doesn't have PMR, but don't let that put you off. We will talk more about this later in this chapter.

For many people, however, having PMR or GCA may only be one of your health challenges[76]. There may be a few barriers to exercising or just generally keeping physically active. In the next section we will look at this in more detail and start to try to suggest some ways to overcome these barriers.

The impact of PMR

If you, or someone you care about, have PMR, you are already an expert in it and fully aware of how life may have changed since developing PMR. However, it's worth taking a moment to consider some other potential coinciding factors might be impacting your life, and the consequences of these.

PMR of course tends to particularly affect older people. But unfortunately, as all of us age, there are also other chronic conditions we may have to live with. For example, some may have joint problems, such as osteoarthritis, or have a heart condition or diabetes. If so, you may already be feeling aches and pains from these too but it probably means you have more than one reason to get more active, so need to be more determined!

You are probably taking steroid medication. Whilst for most people this really helps to manage symptoms of PMR, we have seen in Chapters 3 and 4 that there are side effects and there are now numerous projects looking for alternatives[77]. However, most people who get to read this book will be on steroids for a good while. One of the side effects affecting you may be muscle weakness, also known as steroid myopathy. So, on top of muscles feeling achy from PMR, you may find your muscles feel weak too.

It is understandable when people say they don't feel they have the energy to move or do exercises. However, if we don't, over time this causes other problems, often including more stiffness and pain, and of course our muscles get thinner and weaker. Our bones can also be affected. So, we need to keep moving our bodies and using our muscles in the way they are intended to work.

Take back control!

You need to take back control. However, it isn't that easy. It can feel like a vicious cycle. You try to do some exercise, but it hurts. You rest up (possibly for too long, anxious not to bring back more PMR symptoms) but then feel deflated. You ask yourself why you even tried to be more active in the first place, but at the same time realise you are getting weaker and weaker, stiffer and stiffer over time, mainly due to the inactivity.

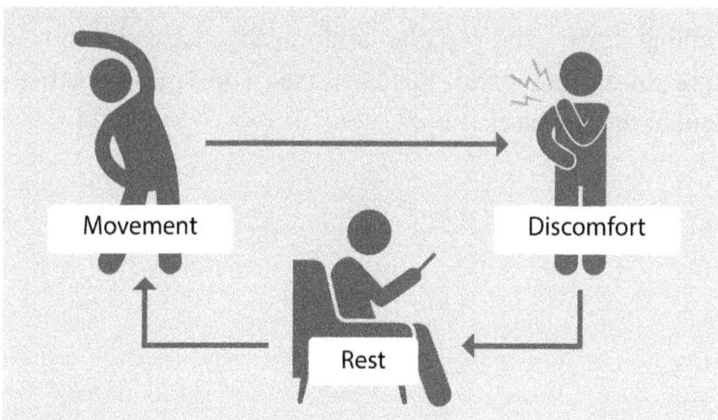

Figure 5; Move, even when it's uncomfortable

You need to try to counteract this. Don't let your PMR dictate your life. Actually, changing your mindset to be more active can really empower you to take back control of how you are living your life with PMR.

Firstly, make an active decision to move, even when it might be a bit uncomfortable, or you just don't feel you have the energy. Thinking beyond what you're immediately feeling, and focussing on the months and years ahead, will help. You are likely to make a good recovery from your PMR, so, it's important to think about the life you want to live when you've recovered from PMR, rather than current symptoms. By focussing on this, and planning how active you want to be, it will help encourage you to keep to your activity plan now.

We know from other inflammatory musculoskeletal conditions that simple stretches (for example for your shoulders or hips) can really help you keep muscles moving and reduce stiffness and muscle aches.

If we keep active and our muscles strong when living with PMR, our balance is likely to be better, we are less likely to fall and therefore less likely to have a fracture/ broken bone, all of which are important to avoid if at all possible. Having a daily activity plan and noting down what you plan to do in advance can be a helpful starting point. But more of this later, (see Top Tips in Section 5 at the end of this chapter).

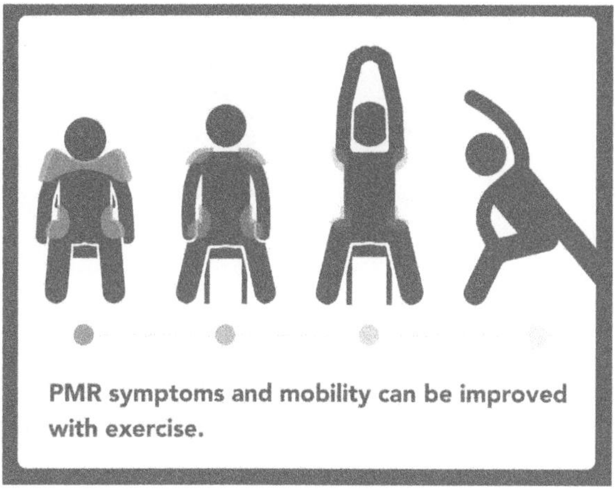

Figure 6: helping symptoms and mobility

Pacing and listening to our bodies to gradually increase activity

So many people say one of the hardest things to learn to do when living with a long-term condition is to get the balance right between moving enough and overdoing it. You may have heard the phrase, it's important to "pace yourself" to make sure you don't overdo it.

Pacing is a way of avoiding a "boom and bust" repetitive cycle. You may recognise this when you are having a better day and fewer PMR symptoms, so you make the most of it, get really busy doing all your jobs. At first, you're really pleased, but then the next day, you recognise, you've overdone it on the better day, and you pay the price for a few days afterwards and just feel exhausted. Does this sound familiar? Well, if you can recognise this pattern, then know you are not alone and take heart. Just by recognising this, you're halfway to solving the problem and avoiding repeating this negative cycle in the future.

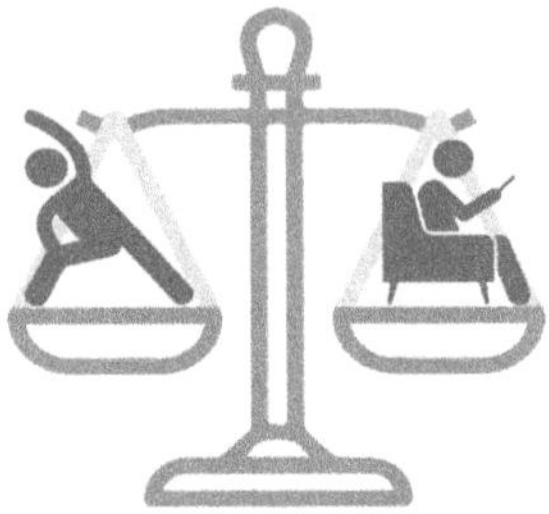

Figure 7: Balancing activity and rest

A big part of pacing is finding the right balance of how much to be active and how much to rest. It's genuinely really hard to get this right and will probably take practice, but it does get easier the more you get good at reading your body's messages to you.

However, while you're finding the balance, don't fall into the trap of being too cautious or protective of yourself. Tempting though it may be to stay in bed, rest up in a chair to avoid movement and possible aches, this is likely to just lead to you getting stiffer and being in more pain. Odd though this may sound, many people describe actually even feeling more tired by "taking it easy."

So, let's break this down a bit and work out what's going on.

Firstly, you have to start to really listen to your body, be more attentive to what it may be telling you. Some of the messages our bodies give us are really subtle, so we sometimes have to "listen" hard! All of us need to remember though that it is usual to feel our bodies more, whether that be our joints or muscles, if we increase our activity levels. So, don't be put off; this is totally normal!

Be patient with yourself. It's often difficult to distinguish what might be our usual aches and pains and general tiredness from everyday life as we get older, from what is actually PMR-related aches and pains. And for most people, finding out is likely to be trial and error.

Does it matter that I'm taking steroids? We also know if someone is taking steroids, some PMR symptoms are masked by the medication, so it can be tricky to work out what's going on. There is no research about this yet, but my experience as a physiotherapist working with people with lots of musculoskeletal conditions has taught me a few things I've summarised below:

1. It is normal for muscles and joints to feel more achy or uncomfortable if you start any new activity or exercise, so don't be put off if you experience this.

2. If pain is worsened by exercises and won't settle after 30-60 mins, then you may have overdone it that day, but don't panic. Just make some small adjustments next time.

3. If your aches don't settle overnight, it's worth being gentler the next day. Try doing half the amount of exercise you did the previous day and see if the pain reoccurs or persists.

4. If the aches are manageable with halving the exercises, then gradually increase little by little over the next week to try to get back to the same amount of exercise as you started doing by 10 days later.

5. Keep listening to your body and ultimately respect pain that is not usual for you. Pain is possibly trying to tell you something about your body, something new to learn. If you are in a lot of discomfort after doing new exercise or activity, give yourself a day off to recover, but then try again the following day.

6. It's important therefore to balance new activities with appropriate rest with exercise, especially if the activities are more strenuous than your usual movements.

7. Try to make sure you get the right amount of sleep. To get the best sleep pattern, many people recommend going to bed at about the same time each night and getting up at similar times

if at all possible. Then if properly rested, you can have more energy to be active.

8. Finally, be prepared to experiment and don't give up. Accept it may be a bit of trial and error. But the most important thing for your long-term health, and to make the best recovery from your PMR, is to keep doing some sort of activity and movement every day.

What should I do if it's really painful?

It is understandable that most of us are afraid when we're in pain. Our natural reaction is to stop moving, sit down and take it easy and maybe even go to bed to rest. However, that is likely to be the worst thing to do if you have PMR. You need to keep to your usual routines as much as possible and keep moving. It will really pay off if you keep your muscles supple and as strong as possible, keep your fitness, even if you're still doing gentler exercise than you'd really want to do.

Nobody is saying this is easy. It really is a balancing act of knowing when to keep moving and when to rest and just take it a bit easier for a day or two. You may get this wrong at times, but the key is to keep trying and keep listening to what your body is trying to tell you.

How many exercises or reps should I do?

This is always a very difficult question to answer because we are all different and we don't have any really good research around this yet. You may have other joint problems or other conditions you are trying to manage. If in doubt, start with few repetitions. You can easily gently build up the number as you feel more confident. If you're doing stretches (which often help reduce feelings of stiffness), try, when you start to feel the stretch, to hold the position for 20-30 seconds. Repeat each stretch between three to five times once a day and then twice a day if you can.

Simple exercises sitting or standing to keep shoulders and hips supple

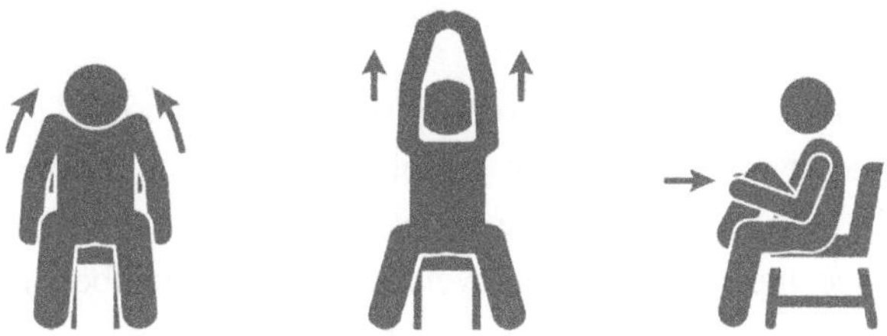

NB: Don't do the hip exercise in the chair if you've been told not to bend beyond 90 degrees (sometimes after hip surgery)

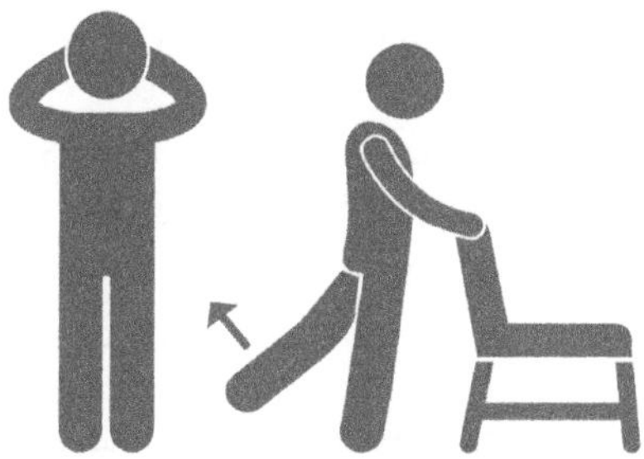

Figure 8: simple standing and sitting exercises

Managing relapse

As you may have already found out, symptoms of PMR are not consistent and the road to recovery can be frustrating and unpredictable. Many people describe times when they feel they are going backwards, and some refer to this as flare, particularly common when you are trying to reduce steroids.

At times like this, it can be so easy to just give up trying to do any exercises or prioritise moving around. This is just the time to remember that even doing small amounts of simple stretching exercises every day, helps keep your body more supple. By keeping moving you'll make it so much easier in the long run to keep physically fit and active.

Prioritising, Pacing and Persevering – the three Ps

So, during a relapse, there are a few things you can do, in addition to remembering to really listen to your body.

1. Prioritise – It's the time to prioritise what you do and don't try to do everything. Some people find making priority lists helpful in planning your week, so you spread out the chores to reduce the likelihood of overdoing it. Remember, like the tortoise and the hare, slow and steady wins the race!

2. Pace – This involves really thinking about and planning your activity in a day and sometimes over a week. If you crack pacing, you'll find your symptoms will be better controlled and you'll be really pleased with the activities you get done.

3. Persevere – This is hard, but you may find using an activity or exercise diary helpful. Just by logging your activity just for a couple of days, you may be surprised that you are actually doing more than you think. And this can be really motivating.

If you decide to try an exercise diary, it needs to include all your everyday activities. Start by thinking about everything you do in your typical day from the time you wake up. You might be surprised as you add it all up. But this may account for why you feel overly tired, especially if you're not balancing your activity out evenly over the week. Don't make this overly laborious. Simple bullet points of what you are doing each day will be sufficient to give you an idea whether some days are typically much busier than others.

Figure 9: Activity diaries

So, make sure to include washing and dressing, time pottering around the house or garden, time doing housework, time out and about shopping, the number of times you climb the stairs, etc. If you only include "proper exercise" (e.g. going to yoga, playing golf or walking the dog for 20 minutes etc.) then you're likely to be underestimating your total daily activity. We could easily almost dismiss all of this everyday moving activity. But if ignored, it could account for why you're feeling exhausted.

Safe and relevant exercises in PMR

In this next section, knowing there are many possible benefits we can get by increasing our daily activity, I suggest some simple exercises, designed with and for people living with PMR, to help you keep supple and flexible, keep you strong, improve your balance and keep you as fit as you can be, whilst lifting your mood in everyday life.

Getting started – preparing to exercise

Being comfortable is vital if you're trying to increase your general activity. So, before you start changing your routines, think about your clothes and shoes. Wearing loose clothes that allow free movement helps. Well-fitting footwear that keeps your feet secure and allows you to have a good firm grip, such as trainers, will also really help you feel more confident as you start to move more. But remember, this doesn't need to cost you loads of money. You don't need to go and buy the latest pair of trainers.

Make a realistic plan and build up activity gradually

I expect many of us can relate to having great New Year intentions to get fitter etc, but actually by January 7th, we're already not keeping to our plan. So, let's keep it real. If you start by changing your routine and trying to just be a bit more active with everyday life, avoid lifts, park a bit further away from store entrances etc, those simple changes will start to make a difference.

But if you're serious and really want to start some exercises, then just start with one or two stretches for your shoulders and a couple for your hips too. Think about where you feel most achy or stiff and start there. In our exercise self-help guide, we have suggested some "beginners" stretches, that can be done daily in sitting or standing as you prefer, (see above), but importantly without any resistance. This is particularly important if you feel you're in a bit of a flare with your PMR.

Progressing from stretching to strengthening and balance exercises

Knowing it's so important for the longer-term to also keep our muscles strong, improve our balance and overall fitness, we also suggest some other "intermediate" and "advanced" exercises to focus more on strength, balance and overall fitness. The images below illustrate what you can do with minimal home weights equipment (e.g. a small bottle of water, or a large potato etc), unless you want to purchase some other kit, such as stretchy resistance bands or hand weights.

Experience and patient feedback suggest a few tips for success:

- Start with a few stretches to warm up before starting with any resistance exercises.

- When beginning any new strengthening exercises, choose just a couple of exercises, (not all) and only try a few repetitions of each initially.
- As few as 5 repetitions, building up to 10 and 20 over a few weeks, should work well for most people. Then you can gradually increase to try them all over a week, so you get a varied programme.
- Begin gently. Some people prefer doing them every other day rather than every day until you know how your body feels doing them.
- Overall, avoid doing more than 10-15 minutes' worth of strengthening exercises in one day initially. That way you should avoid feeling too achy afterwards

Keeping a diary, noting how many repetitions you have done and importantly, how you feel after your exercises that day and then the next day, (including your overall mood) might be really helpful and encouraging.

Before you start any of these exercises, think about improving your posture. If seated, sit upright, but be comfortable. If standing, stand tall, shoulders back and stomach in.

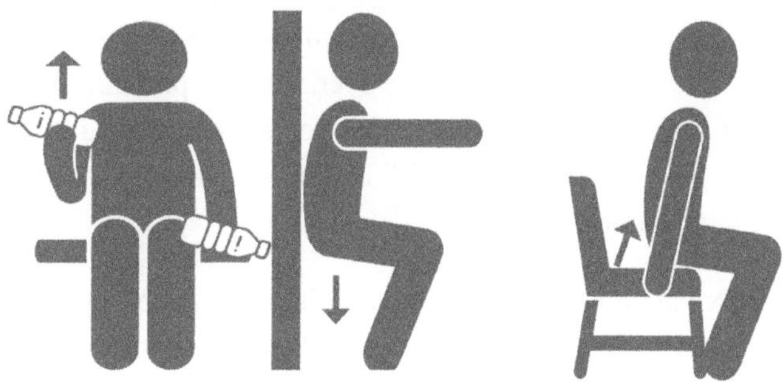

Keep your back straight as you slowly stand up and down

Figure 10: Strengthening exercises for arms and legs

- Wall squats – lower yourself slowly, sliding down a supporting wall until you feel your leg muscles are beginning to work hard. You may only want to hold this for 10 seconds before standing upright again. Try to repeat three times and over the next few weeks try and hold the squat position for longer building up to 60 seconds if you can.

- For the repeated sitting to standing exercise, you are trying to move like you're in slow motion. This makes your muscles work a lot harder, but it is still gentle to do. Start doing five repetitions once or twice a day and gradually build the number up so you can do 10 repetitions.

For these muscle strengthening exercises, it's best to do all of them slowly. Avoid any jerky movements and try and keep your movements smooth. It may take a couple of weeks, but your muscles will start getting stronger. You might notice this in your walking or climbing stairs or getting in and out of a low chair, all of which may start to get easier.

Exercise to improve balance and reduce the risk of falls

The good news is that both these leg strengthening exercises above will not only work to get you feeling stronger, but they will also help your balance. Having strong leg muscles is really important if we lose our balance because they will be able to quickly work to reduce the chance of us falling over. As you probably know, the risk of a fracture following a fall for anyone taking steroids is greater, so if we can avoid a fall by keeping strong and active, this is a big advantage.

If you've already had a fall though, there are people who can help you avoid having another one. So, it may be worth telling your doctor or practice nurse. It may be worth someone doing a falls assessment with you especially as you have PMR[78].

Improving overall fitness and mood

Several of the strengthening exercises, if you do enough of them, might make you a bit short of breath, so they will help you get fitter over time. But there are also some simple home exercises you can do to will really improve your fitness, and also give a sense of wellbeing and achievement.

For example, if you have stairs or even one back step, you might want to try some "step ups" or go back to the sitting to standing exercise above and just speed it up, which will increase your heart rate. All of us should be trying to do at least 30 minutes' worth of exercise to make ourselves feel a bit short of breath five times a week or the equivalent, so 150 minutes of moderately intensive exercise over a week[79].

As with all exercise, we need to start gently. If you're not used to any exercise, five or ten minutes of the exercises below will be a great start, or maybe just doing some walking on the spot, or faster walking than normal. Then, when this feels OK you can gradually add in these other fitness exercises. Having breaks is fine, so it may suit you better to do ten minutes of exercise three times over a day instead of one block. Remember, every bit of extra exercise you do will make a difference over time.

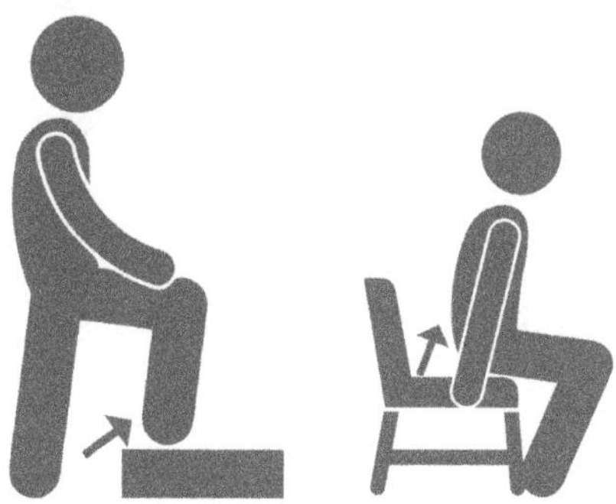

Figure 11: Exercises for fitness

Top Tips for being active with PMR

There is a lot we could talk further about, but this chapter boils down to some simple key messages. The following points sum it up.

1. Learn to listen to your body
2. Try to have a regular activity routine, but adjust exercises when necessary
3. Balance activity with rest
4. Be alert to symptoms returning
5. Don't give up and expect some ups and downs
6. When in doubt, keep moving

No matter how inactive you usually are, you can make a difference and take some control of your PMR by making small changes in everyday life and move a bit more. There are multiple health benefits to doing more physical activity and it needn't be expensive or time consuming. Many people describe exercise easing their PMR aches and stiffness. And most people describe having more energy for everyday life and just feeling in a better mood when they are more active. So, what are you waiting for?

Fortunately, the long-term outlook with PMR is good. Most people do recover from this after a few years, so, even though we age whilst living with PMR, we still need to keep active in between and get our post-PMR-body ready for an active older age! Good luck!

Postscript: advice for those who were very active before PMR or GCA

Many thanks to Anne for sharing her professional expertise, experience and empathy. If you were very active before developing PMR or GCA, as I was, this is often the hardest adjustment. I had been a long-distance runner, and I took the change very hard, as though I had become an old and disabled person overnight. I had 'used' running as a way of mitigating my stress levels at work, and so I felt, in giving up exercise, I had lost an important safety valve in my daily life.

Walking, and later, cycling, proved a big help during my years with PMR. A drop in stamina and strength such as I felt is very common, even when motivation is still there. That doesn't mean you have to give up what you enjoy, but it does mean changing how you approach it.

Pam, in her 70s with GCA, a keen cyclist, tells us how GCA impacted on her activities:

> *"Before my GCA diagnosis, aged 70, I would easily cycle 100 miles a week, so 5,000 miles a year and happily keep pace with women 20 years my junior – even outstripping them on hills!*
>
> *"My first concern was - would I be able to keep up this level of cycling? The steroids only added to my apparent level of fitness and four months later I was happily flying up Mallorcan mountains with no apparent ill effects immediately afterwards. However, a few days later I had my first flare, and I felt this could well have been self-inflicted.*
>
> *"For the last couple of years, I have halved my mileage and scaled back on elevation. Naturally this has affected my cardio fitness immensely. Worse still it has a profound effect on me psychologically as I am no longer able to ride in the same way with friends, take part in sportives, attack the mountains or even do touring holidays in the same way.*
>
> *"My frustration is that I have the energy to cycle, but my body seems to call time periodically and there are no clear signals why it has. I have had two subsequent flares and the last has left me lacking in confidence about getting on my*

bike. Two and a half years down the road, I definitely notice that I am tired the day after a really short 15-mile ride. But if I wasn't afraid of the consequences, I would definitely be doing more mileage and more hill climbing!"

"I have tried strength training, try to do more walking and go regularly to Pilates as a way of mitigating my declining fitness, but it is the loss of cardio fitness that disappoints me most. I really wish there was more research into physical exercise and GCA."

You, like me, may well be gobsmacked at Pam's level of cycling, even now with GCA. One thing that shines out of her story is her will and motivation to carry on being an athlete. She is proof against all the tired stereotypes of older people "taking it easy".

The secret is Anne's advice about pacing: finding a level your body can cope with and gradually building from there. Many people find they can only get back to about half of their previous level, at least for a time.

8 Support is out there

However independent we want to be, we all need support, to break the isolation that having PMR and GCA can thrust upon us. I've told the story earlier of my experience of feeling blocked as I was trying to taper the steroids. After that, I did start to take a more active role in my condition, and found out about Patient Experience, an early patient website, where I made contact with other people suffering from PMR who understood what I was going through, because they were going through it too. I began to understand that I did not simply have a condition affecting my muscles. I had an illness coursing through my whole body, affecting every part of my organism in one way or another. And the bits unaffected by my illness – well, they were affected by the medication.

This was the point at which I started to look for the patients' support organisation that could tell me more about PMR and answer my many questions. And when I didn't manage to find it, I reached out to others on Patient Experience to ask if anyone was interested in helping me start a charity. I set up the email address pmrfighters@gmail.com and waited. It didn't take long for four people to get in touch, all as frustrated and fired up as I was. Looking back, I can see I was probably over the worst of the illness to have the drive to begin. But at the same time, I felt trapped in a situation where what should have been a smooth steady taper was like the up and down zigzag of a dragon's back. That was in 2008.

Thankfully, there are now several sources of support available. In England, PMRGCAuk and its affiliated support groups, and in Scotland, PMR and GCA Scotland, are providing helpline services and sending out information packs to people who are newly diagnosed and those some way into treatment. There is a vibrant PMRGCAuk online community on the HealthUnlocked platform, and people are able to connect with one another in ways only dreamed of a few years ago.

PMRGCAuk Helpline

The first thing bringing people together to form the group that would become PMRGCAuk was we all agreed there should be a helpline. Since then, many of us (but by no means all) have got used to texting and typing, but there is nothing to beat the sound of another human voice when we are feeling alone and vulnerable. PMR and GCA patients have felt the shock and bewilderment of being told we have a disease nobody else has even heard of. The founders of the charity wanted there to be help at the end of the phone for anybody, whether they needed information, reassurance, or just a listening ear.

We registered two phone numbers: 0300 111 5090, and 0300 999 5090. The 0300 was a standard free to call code. The 111 and 999 were a kind of homage to emergency services, and the 5090 reflected the fact that people between 50 and 90 get diagnosed with PMR and GCA. There was talk about using the 999 number for the helpline, but one school of thought was it was too alarmist, and so we opted for 111 to be the helpline number. And it has been in place for 15 years.

I asked Fiona Johnson, the current Chair of Trustees, to update me on how the helpline is going. It's still an important part of the charity's support system. Not everyone likes to be online, and many people still prefer to talk to a live person rather than type on a keyboard.

Nowadays, the helpline receives two or three calls a day. People can call for all sorts of reasons, but they tend to fall into three main types. The first is people who have only just been diagnosed, and who want more information. Just under half of callers fall into this category. Sometimes they are panicking slightly. Often their GPs have printed out some (barely adequate) information in the surgery and sent them home to read through it, and with luck they have found the helpline number at the bottom. There are still delays for people who are suspected of having GCA - they don't always get to see a specialist on the same day, by any means - they need advice and information on what to watch out for while they are waiting.

Advisers can give these callers information (but not so much that they are overloaded, because they need time to absorb it) and some reassurance that the chances are they will start feeling better soon. There is a handy information pack sent out to these people for them to go through in their own time. It includes the most up-to-date leaflet from ArthritisUK, an umbrella charity for a host of inflammatory conditions. The information pack is available both in hard copy and an electronic version via the PMRGCAuk website, and in the year 2023-24 more than 1500 were requested.

Roger, a keen golfer in his 70s, says:

> *"I called the helpline and felt so much better afterwards. I can't tell you how much difference it makes to speak to someone who has had the condition, who knows what it's like and can share their own experiences. I was directed to a paper on the website by a top rheumatologist. It gave me the tools to go back to my doctor and discuss things like dosage."*

The second type of caller (about 40%) is people who are quite a long way into their PMR or GCA journey, say two to four years, and are having trouble tapering. GPs and information leaflets tend to give the impression that lowering the dose and coming off prednisolone is a fairly smooth and trouble-free process. But not everyone feels ready or confident about it at the start and then relapses will set them back and damage their confidence further. Many find it really hard, and then they start to wonder if they are the only people who are suffering like this. Some can even start to blame themselves for not being "good" patients. In this scenario, the helpline volunteer can reassure and help the patient rehearse the conversation they want to have with their doctor.

Some people are being offered methotrexate and need to talk through their questions and concerns with someone who is both a lay person and knowledgeable at the same time, a person who can help them make up their own mind.

Another group of callers is those, often in their 70s or 80s, who have been stricken with PMR or GCA on top of other long-term conditions. They may already be taking complicated mixes of drugs and are worried about the way in which both their 'new' illness, and the prednisolone, might affect their pre-existing conditions. For volunteers, it can be a challenge because they have to explain why they cannot give individual clinical advice. However, most people find it really helpful just to share their concerns with somebody who is a good listener and understands what they have been going through. Average calls last 15-20 minutes and callers will never be rushed. Almost everyone says, at the end of a call, that it was great to talk with somebody who has, or has had, this peculiar illness.

Fiona notices a certain difference between male and female callers, in that many of the men who phone the helpline are struggling with work-related issues. About one in four callers is a man. They may be being impacted by the physical effects of PMR and the consequences for their earnings. They may be professionals who have been very fit and active previously and are suffering psychologically because a) they're not used to being in pain and b) having a chronic rheumatic illness wasn't part of their "script" in middle age. Fortunately, information can often help such individuals, because knowing what is happening and what to expect can help them manage their feelings. Apparently, repeat callers are almost always women, for some reason.

In earlier chapters we've referred to ways you can prepare yourself for a conversation with your GP or rheumatologist, and how to plan, getting your facts and questions ready so you don't forget anything or end up feeling bamboozled. Remember, if you feel you could benefit from a listening ear at this stage, the helpline is there for you.

The volunteers on the helpline do not have any particular qualifications but do receive training from a professional, and there are strict guidelines. Several volunteers have managed helplines or related services in previous careers. Some helpline volunteers are also busy organising support groups. The charity is always on the lookout for people to join the team. Do you have some experience of counselling, or another role where you have to use high level listening skills? Do you have a few hours or a few days when you could be at home to take calls or deal with messages? Would you like to help people in the same boat as yourself? If the answer is yes, please get in touch with the PMRGCAuk office number, 0300 999 5090. They would be so happy to hear from you!

Support groups

The first support group in England, as far as we know, was set up near Ipswich by Jennifer Nott in 2004. Jean Miller had already got a group going in Scotland. This was closely followed by a group in Southend, linked to Prof. Dasgupta and his team. Over the years, a network has developed across Great Britain, every group being created and nurtured by a volunteer, often a PMR or GCA patient themselves, driven by an urge to share and help others. In 2024, there were 36 groups in England and Wales. Scotland is served by PMR&GCA Scotland. Groups sometimes meet online, especially since the pandemic when we got used to meeting via our phone and computer screens.

Most of the groups meet regularly, although not too often. As you can imagine, it is quite a demanding thing to organise a group when you are perhaps not feeling too well yourself. All support groups are patient-led and owe their existence to the efforts and energies of determined PMR and GCA sufferers who want to help other people in a similar position to themselves.

One legendary trailblazer is the late Mavis Smith, who famously travelled from Gateshead to London in a taxi in 2008 to attend the meeting for the formation of PMRGCAuk. Mavis, Pam and Margaret were three northern ladies who ran a network in the north-east for more than a decade. Since we lost them, it has become a concern that there are significantly more support groups in southern England than in the north.

Groups have a range of activities, from guest speakers such as the local consultant rheumatologist, to movement sessions with physiotherapists, and contributions from herbalists or other alternative therapists. Clinicians find the time they spend attending a group meeting to speak is a great way to give out information and learn from patients. A group situation can often increase and improve overall levels of communication. I do believe it is good for consultants to see their patients outside the clinical setting, to see them as whole people with families and a place in the community. An essential feature, though, is the support, solidarity, understanding and acceptance people with PMR and GCA can share with each other. In plenty of group sessions, members just meet up to chat, share experiences and cheer each other up.

Successful as the network of groups is, there are still huge gaps around the UK, such as in the north, and the West Midlands. As with the helpline, PMRGCAuk is always on the lookout for people who can help set up and run groups.

Shirley, who ran the Surrey group, put it like this:

> *"The spur I needed to set up the Group, as a long term sufferer of PMR/GCA, was not only remembering the many unanswered questions about both the illness and the subsequent treatment*

that ran around in my head during the early days, but most of all the overwhelming feeling of isolation which only ended when I came across a group of other sufferers online."

No doubt, PMRGCAuk is no different from other health charities in finding its network of support groups is valuable for sufferers of chronic health conditions; but some things make our groups amazing. The first is that the average age of members of PMRGCAuk is about 76. It is quite something for a person who has PMR or GCA themselves, perhaps well into their 60s, to set up and manage a group for other people, and for older people to make huge efforts to travel many miles in some cases to their regular group meeting. One incentive is that group members get to meet people at different stages of their illness. Those newly diagnosed can learn what may be facing them in the future (good and not-so-good!) and those further on in their journey can see how far they have come. In a survey, seven out of ten group members said that being part of the group made them feel more optimistic about their prospects for recovery. This just shows how important it is to reduce the sense of isolation.

If you're interested in joining a support group, PMRGCAuk can point you in the right direction. And they also have lots of experience and expertise to help you if you fancy setting one up in your own area.

HealthUnlocked - the patient support forum

One day, around 2012, our office team of two, myself and assistant Nadia, working on building PMRGCAuk, was approached by a mysterious organisation calling itself HealthUnlocked. They wanted to offer us a space on their website for PMR and GCA patients to contact each other and share information, advice and support. We were circumspect. Why did we need another website? We already had one. There were already a couple of forums. What was the motivation for the founders of HealthUnlocked (who were doctors, by the way)?

We decided to give it a go for a trial period. Fourteen years on, over 22,000 people have registered on the HealthUnlocked forum. It has become not only a massive source of support and information for patients, but also an important bank of data and patient experience.

People can post questions about any aspect of their experience with PMR and/or GCA, and other members can give advice, information or encouragement. Members can also blog about their experience, which, besides being interesting for other people living with the conditions, makes them feel they are not on their own.

Being a member of the web forum is great for people who have complex health conditions running alongside their PMR or GCA. For example, people with heart conditions predating their PMR or GCA, who have concerns about the cocktail of medications they are taking. They can almost always get a response to their questions from somebody who has either been in the same position or knows something about it. Many of the members say they get more information from the forum than from anywhere else. "Fressia" says,

> *"I have found this website so informative and a comfort to know other PMR sufferers are having exactly the same problems as myself."*

If you would like to contact other people with PMR or GCA, join - it's easy! Just go to healthunlocked.com, sign up, and search for polymyalgia rheumatica or giant cell arteritis.

Access to the forum is free, but of course, depends on PMRGCAuk resources, staff and volunteers. Just imagine, if everyone on the forum joined the charity, that would generate nearly half a million pounds for raising awareness, lobbying and supporting research.

Internet forums are becoming a huge bank of knowledge and experience. Gaining support from other patients is, however, not without its issues. We have to remember at all times that our fellow forum members, and support group members for that matter, are not medically qualified. This, you might say, is actually a benefit, especially if you have had negative experiences with your GP or consultant. However, it can be risky to accept advice from unqualified people on issues such as a personalised steroid dose or a tapering regime. We constantly need to be monitoring our own actions and reactions, for example asking ourselves, "Why would I trust a lay person I have never met and who knows nothing about me, to give me advice about my condition, more than I would trust my doctor?" I would always recommend sharing the information and ideas gleaned from the forum with your doctor before making changes. This is particularly important when it comes to adjusting your steroid dose.

HealthUnlocked is staffed by people who really know what they are talking about, who have spent years learning as much about PMR and GCA as they possibly can, and who are trusted by PMRGCAuk. We can't say the same about Facebook, for example. There are now several groups on FB for people with PMR and GCA, with no apparent affiliations. This is just testimony to how so many people feel completely at sea when they are trying to manage their condition. Especially when they are feeling unwell, anxious and unhappy.

My caveat about taking what people on Facebook say as gospel truth is that many folks have their own agendas, or they have a pet idea about what caused their illness or what is curing them. This is particularly the case when it comes to diet, when all kinds of ideas about wonder anti-inflammation diets are spread around. "A nutritionist told me this", "A naturopathic doctor told me that" may be interesting, but not authoritative. I've seen people say things like "I'm taking 10mg pred at the moment. I've found that cutting out carbs completely has totally dealt with my pain." I can't help feeling that there's a blind spot there!

"Don" on Facebook put it better than I could:

> *"I've seen and read many 'I have the answer' fill-in-the-blank cures for this disease. You can go down various rabbit holes with no real answers. I appreciate people want to find an answer, but if it was as simple as what some folks present, and their cure worked, it would be mainstream news in a heartbeat. Until then, I will continue to pray for a true and lasting cure."*

The unmet need

Of course, we would all love there to be a cure, but until then, researchers around the world are working on answering some of the more slippery questions posed by PMR and GCA. It is worth focusing for a while on areas of research that promise to improve the patient experience. We can then understand the need for patient-advocacy organisations like PMRGCAuk to put resources into fostering research and disseminating new findings.

The PMR Paradox study, based in Leeds, arose from a tantalising conundrum. As PMR and GCA are more prevalent in Scandinavian countries and in areas of the USA with high numbers of people of Scandi heritage, one would expect there would be a concentration of cases in the north of England, and in Scotland, where there are more people with Scandi heritage in their DNA.

But rates of diagnosis are actually lower than in the south of England. What's going on? Is there under diagnosis in the north? Is there over-diagnosis in the south? Could it be a combination of both? And what are the factors contributing to this situation?

The paradox study has opened up dialogue about a whole range of aspects of the patient experience, and generated lots of directions for future research[80].

One theme that came out strongly was the sense of isolation many people feel if their PMR or GCA doesn't follow the conventional course outlined in the guidelines. If you are relatively young (under 55), or have normal blood markers, or a non-standard response to steroid therapy, having PMR or GCA can feel incredibly isolating, even if you have access to online information and support. If your doctor regularly gives out verbal or nonverbal signals they themselves are not confident of the diagnosis, it can be very unsettling. You can start to wish you had more standard signs and symptoms just to make the doctor feel better! But it's not your job to make the doctor feel better.

Here's a rundown of key areas for progress that Vanessa and I hope to see in the years ahead, which will improve patient experience and outcomes.

Improving service provision for PMR

Delayed diagnosis or Misdiagnosis

As we have seen, PMR can mimic other conditions, such as RA, malignancy, and infections. As no definitive test exists, diagnosis follows a process of excluding other conditions, and this increases variability in care. GPs need more awareness of differential diagnoses. We need improved early referral protocols for atypical or steroid-resistant cases. Failing that, a standardised diagnostic pathway for GPs to follow, and shared care protocols between GPs and rheumatologists.

Inadequate Steroid Management and Monitoring

GPs often lack confidence in monitoring cases and tapering steroids. Side effects are often not proactively monitored. There is a lack of consistency in bone protection, DEXA scanning, and patient education on steroid risks. And, as routine, inclusion of bone health assessment, blood glucose checks, and steroid toxicity reviews are required.

Relapse Recognition and Management

Fifty percent of patients flare during tapering, but guidance on how to manage relapse is inconsistent. Misidentification may lead to unnecessary escalation of steroids or missed GCA. Patients might be driven to self-medicate. What's needed are clear, national relapse management protocols, and improved use of inflammatory markers and, potentially, imaging in complex cases.

Improving GCA provision

GCA is a medical emergency — yet service provision across the UK still shows major gaps affecting outcomes such as sight loss, vascular complications, and quality of life. Key areas of unmet need include:

Emergency Pathways and Fast Diagnosis

Best practice needs to be standard for everyone. The sooner people can be diagnosed, the more likely that sight loss can be avoided and people can get the correct diagnosis. There is now plenty of evidence fast-track pathways work and save money. Every hospital should have a team of technicians or clinicians trained up to do temporal and axillary artery ultrasound examinations, ending the postcode lottery. Surgical biopsies as a first line test should be a thing of the past.

Access to Biologics

The limit set by NICE for the provision of tocilizumab to patients with relapsing GCA was a kind of political (with a small p) compromise, between NICE and Roche, the licensee pharmaceutical company that made the first tocilizumab called Actemra. The experts at Roche must have had their fingers crossed hoping the vast majority of patients taking TCZ would be free of GCA within the year. There is now ample evidence though that once people hit the deadline and come off TCZ, a significant proportion start relapsing again.

We really need a new campaign to extend this one-year limit so patients can fully benefit from the new drugs. The key point being, without them, patients would be taking much higher cumulative doses of steroids, which would be far more harmful. NICE usually review their guidance three years after publication, which would have been 2021, so it's long overdue. At the time of writing in early 2026, NICE are still making up their mind about whether to fund upadacitinib in GCA, and how long to fund it for. Their decision will likely lay the path for other biologic and targeted therapies in GCA. The fight to allow these drugs for PMR in the NHS has not yet begun. Another reason to join and support PMRGCAuk!

Become a member of PMRGCAuk

For just £22 a year at the time of writing, you can become a member of the support charity at the heart of patient representation in PMR and GCA. At the end of March 2024, PMRGCAuk had 1600 registered members, of whom 440 had registered during the previous year. People tend to let their membership lapse once they recover, but almost half of the membership have been members for three or more years.

As one of the smaller charities in the UK focusing on health conditions, and conditions affecting overwhelmingly older people at that, PMRGCAuk faces particular challenges in attracting the funding needed to resource its activities. Paid employees can be counted on the fingers of one hand, and you can be confident all of your membership fees and any donations go direct to supporting the charity's work. A proportion of the proceeds from this book goes to help the charity, but please do a little more and become a member. In return you get access to special resources and events. It's really worth every penny!

In 2017, PMRGCAuk conducted, with a group of academics based at Keele University, a questionnaire survey of members, aimed at establishing patients' priorities for support[81]. It was striking that 76% of the people who responded cited being on steroids and trying to reduce steroids as their biggest area of need for support. This is important, especially as there is very little in the way of an evidence base to inform the support they should be getting from their doctors.

This leads on to another important role for a charity like PMRGCAuk; representing patients to the medical world, to improve education and awareness. It's as crucial for clinicians to understand the patient experience and patient concerns as it is for patients to understand about their conditions. A patient charity provides the perfect channel for this to happen.

And to sum up, in the words of a member of PMRGCAuk:

> *"I found it difficult to understand what had happened to me, how my life had changed so suddenly, and you made me feel less alone and more able to sort myself out."*

A life-changing gift

Having PMR in my 50s was a kind of gift in a way. One I would not have chosen, don't get me wrong, but a gift, nonetheless. The restrictions on mobility, the pain and discomfort that slowed me down, gave me insights into the daily experience of people older and frailer than myself. I was a better daughter for that. I realised how intolerant the world in general is towards people who have physical disabilities, and how challenging the mundane activities of normal daily life can be for people with chronic health problems. I vowed I would hold on to this memory and use it to make myself more patient and more tolerant of others.

Working with PMRGCAuk has also been a gift, bringing me into contact with hundreds of wonderful people, many of whom are fighting their battle against ill health on their own, many of whom have other serious conditions along with their GCA or PMR. If you are one of them and are reading this, please accept my thanks for all you have taught me.

By 2016 I had been chair and *de facto* director since 2010, and after six years as a trustee I had continued to work with the charity. I published the second edition of this book, writing the main part of the manuscript in a frenzy of just a few weeks.

When my parents became so frail that they needed constant care and attention, it was time for me to turn my attention and energies to the family. Since then, for years, I had remained a member of PMRGCAuk, but at arms' length, and was frankly daunted by the prospect of updating the book. Vanessa was the perfect co-author to give me the motivation I needed, and of course this edition could not have been created without her fantastic knowledge and commitment. I have learned so much from our collaboration and am in awe of her commitment to her patients.

And so here I am, ten years on, in my mid-70s, picking up where I left off, with new colleagues (and, happily, some old ones), new friends and new knowledge to get my head around. It's really been a privilege.

Signing off

We have now come to the end of our journey through PMR and GCA, and how they impact your lives. We hope it has helped to make things clearer, and perhaps a little less worrying too, and that you don't feel so alone. We also hope it gives you some idea about what is possible, and what could be just on the horizon for future developments. We want you to know that there are people who care very deeply about polymyalgia rheumatica and giant cell arteritis – enough to dedicate their careers to them. And by extension, to you too.

You have the measure of that dragon. Whether your story is just beginning, or has been going a while, you have more ahead of you. As well as taking this book with you as your companion and champion to refer to from time to time, please accept our very best wishes for your full recovery.

Kate Gilbert and Vanessa Quick.

Appendix A: Treat to Target

Extracted from Dejaco, C *et al.* (2024) Treat to target recommendations in giant cell arteritis and polymyalgia rheumatica, *Annals of the Rheumatic Diseases,* vol.83, issue 1. https://ard.bmj.com/content/83/1/48.info.

Overarching principles

Clinical management of GCA and PMR should be driven by the awareness that they are closely interrelated conditions in a common spectrum of inflammatory diseases and can occur separately, simultaneously, or in temporal sequence to each other

GCA is a medical emergency because of the imminent risk of sight loss and other ischaemic events and, therefore, requires immediate treatment; management usually requires multidisciplinary collaboration.

Patients should be offered access to information about GCA and PMR, including clinical disease features, patient-reported outcomes, potential complications, treatment-related benefits and risks, as well as relevant comorbidities.

Management of GCA and PMR should be based on shared decision-making between the informed patient and the physician.

Treatment of GCA and PMR should aim at maximising health-related quality of life through control of symptoms, preventing disease-related damage and minimising treatment-related adverse consequences, taking relevant comorbidities into account.

Specific recommendations

The treatment target of GCA and PMR should be remission; remission is the absence of clinical symptoms and systemic inflammation.

Treatment of GCA should also aim to prevent tissue ischaemia and vascular damage.

Treatment selection in GCA and PMR should be based on disease severity and activity, presence of relevant comorbidities and potential predictors of outcome; treatment should be modified as needed during follow-up.

Comorbidities may influence the assessment of the treatment target and should be considered before modifying treatment.

Once remission is reached, it should be maintained with the minimal effective dose of medication: drug free remission may be achieved in a proportion of patients.

Disease activity in GCA and PMR should be monitored regularly, as frequently as every 1–4 weeks until remission has been achieved, and at longer monitoring intervals (e.g., between 3 and 6 months) in patients in stable remission on therapy; monitoring of patients off therapy should be discussed on an individual basis.

Appendix B: Glossary of terms

aneurysm	An abnormal bulging or ballooning of a blood vessel wall caused by weakening of the vessel, which can enlarge over time and carries a small risk of rupture.
arteritis	Inflammation of an artery that can narrow or damage the blood vessel, reducing blood flow to tissues and organs.
biopsy	A small sample of tissue taken to test for abnormalities.
bisphosphonates	Medicines that help strengthen bones by slowing bone loss, reducing the risk of fractures.
blepharitis	Inflammation of the edges of the eyelids, causing redness, irritation, crusting and a gritty or burning sensation in the eyes
bursitis	Inflammation of a small fluid-filled sac near a joint, which normally helps reduce friction, causing pain and stiffness around the affected area.
claudication	A cramping aching pain, heaviness or fatigue, in the muscles, that comes on with use and gets better with rest.
CRP test	A blood test measuring C-reactive protein, which rises in the blood when there is inflammation in the body and helps assess disease activity or response to treatment.
cytokines	Proteins released by cells that act as chemical messengers, helping to control inflammation and coordinate the body's immune response.
DEXA scan	A specialised X-ray scan that measures bone strength and helps assess the risk of osteoporosis and fractures.
DMARD	Disease-modifying antirheumatic drug
ESR	A blood test called the erythrocyte sedimentation rate that measures how quickly red blood cells settle in a tube, which can indicate the presence of inflammation in the body.
fibromyalgia	A long-term condition causing widespread muscle and joint pain, fatigue, poor sleep, and heightened sensitivity to pain, without ongoing inflammation or tissue damage.
GPSD	GCA PMR Spectrum Disorder
glucocorticoids	A group of steroid medicines that reduce inflammation and suppress the immune system, commonly used to treat conditions such as PMR and GCA. Examples include prednisolone, prednisone, and intravenous methylprednisolone.
granulomatosis	Inflammation characterised by clusters of immune cells forming small nodules in tissues, often as part of a chronic inflammatory or immune condition.
inflammation	A protective response of the immune system that normally helps fight infection or injury, but in autoimmune and inflammatory diseases becomes overactive and misdirected,

	leading to ongoing pain, swelling, heat, stiffness, and tissue damage.
interleukins	Immune system messenger proteins that help control inflammation and can drive symptoms when overactive.
ischaemia/ischaemic	A restriction in blood supply to any tissue, muscle group, or organ of the body, causing a shortage of oxygen that is needed for cellular metabolism.
leflunomide	A disease-modifying medicine that dampens the immune system to reduce inflammation and help control autoimmune conditions.
MRI scan	A magnetic resonance imaging scan, which uses strong magnets and radio waves to create detailed pictures of the inside of the body without using X-rays.
methotrexate	A disease-modifying medicine that reduces immune system overactivity to control inflammation in autoimmune conditions such as PMR, GCA, and inflammatory arthritis.
myopathy	A condition in which the muscles are weakened or damaged, leading to loss of strength and difficulty with everyday movements.
neutrophils	A type of white blood cell which helps fight infection.
pectoral girdle	See shoulder girdle.
pelvic girdle	The ring of bone protecting the lower internal organs, and formed of fused bones, the ilium, the ischium and the pubis.
peripheral neuropathy	Peripheral neuropathy is damage to the nerves outside the brain and spine that can cause tingling, numbness, pain, or weakness, usually in the hands and feet.
PET scan	A positron emission tomography scan, which uses a small amount of radioactive tracer to highlight areas of inflammation in the body.
phenotype	Any observable characteristic or trait of a disease, such as morphology, development, biochemical or physiological properties, or behaviour.
polyangiitis	Inflammation affecting many small blood vessels throughout the body, which can disrupt blood flow and damage organs and tissues.
polymyalgic symptoms	Widespread muscle pain and stiffness, often affecting the shoulders, neck, and hips, particularly on waking or after rest, which may be due to PMR but can occur in other conditions too.
prednisolone	A steroid medicine that reduces inflammation and suppresses the immune system, commonly used to treat PMR, GCA, and other inflammatory conditions.
prednisone	A steroid medicine that is converted to prednisolone in the liver. It's favoured in the States over prednisolone due to clinical tradition and familiarity; the difference between the two drugs is rarely important unless someone has severe liver disease.

proximal	Referring to something closer to the centre of the body or point of origin, such as the shoulders or hips rather than the hands or feet.
rheumatology	Rheumatology is a branch of medicine devoted to the diagnosis and management of disorders whose common feature is inflammation in the bones, muscles, joints, and internal organs.
shoulder girdle	The shoulder girdle or pectoral girdle is the set of bones that connects to the arm on each side. In humans, it consists of the clavicle and scapula.
spectrum	A spectrum disorder is a disorder that includes a range of linked conditions. The different elements of a spectrum either have a similar appearance or are thought to be caused by the same underlying mechanism.
tapering	The process of gradually lessening the dosage of steroids, eventually reaching or approaching zero.
temporal	Connected to the temple area at the side of the head.
tenosynovitis	Inflammation of the lining around a tendon, causing pain, swelling, and difficulty moving the affected joint.
tocilizumab	A biologic medicine that blocks the inflammatory messenger interleukin 6, helping reduce inflammation and steroid dependence in conditions such as GCA and PMR.
tomography	A technique for displaying a representation of a cross section through a human body or other solid object.
ultrasound	sound or other vibrations having an ultrasonic frequency, particularly as used in medical imaging.
vasculitis	A group of conditions that damage blood vessels by causing inflammation or swelling. Vasculitis can affect any size and type of blood vessel (arteries and veins), anywhere in the body.

References

1. Ameer, F. and McNeil J. Polymyalgia rheumatica: clinical update. Australian Family Physician. 2014;43(6):373-376.
2. Dasgupta B, et al. BSR and BHPR guidelines for the management of polymyalgia rheumatica. Rheumatology (Oxford). 2010;49(1):186–190.
3. Dejaco C. et al. 2015. 2015 recommendations for the management of polymyalgia rheumatica: a European League Against Rheumatism/American College of Rheumatology collaboration initiative, Annals of the Rheumatic Diseases. 2015;74(10):1799-1807.
4. Dasgupta B, et al. BSR and BHPR guidelines for the management of giant cell arteritis. Rheumatology (Oxford). 2010;49(8):1594–1597.
5. British Society for Rheumatology. What is rheumatology? [Internet]. London: British Society for Rheumatology; 2022 [cited 2025 Oct 24]. Available from: https://www.rheumatology.org.uk/what-is-rheumatology
6. Castañeda S, et al. Advances in the treatment of giant cell arteritis. J Clin Med. 2022;11(6):1588. doi:10.3390/jcm11061588.
7. Dejaco C, et al. The spectrum of giant cell arteritis and polymyalgia rheumatica: revisiting the concept of the disease. Rheumatology (Oxford). 2017;56(4):506–515. doi:10.1093/rheumatology/kew273.
8. Cowley S, et al. Should all patients with polymyalgia rheumatica have a vascular ultrasound assessment? Ann Rheum Dis. 2024;83(8):961-964. doi:10.1136/ard-2024-225650.
9. HealthUnlocked, PMRGCAuk community [Internet]. Available from: https://healthunlocked.com/pmrgcauk.
10. Chatzidionysiou K. Rheumatic disease and artistic creativity. Mediterranean Journal of Rheumatology. 2019;30(2):103–109. doi:10.31138/mjr.30.2.103.
11. Leung J. et al. 2019. Management of polymyalgia rheumatica in older people, Journal of Pharmacy Practice and Research. 2019;49(5):493–500.
12. Dasgupta B, et al. 2012 Provisional classification criteria for polymyalgia rheumatica: a European League Against Rheumatism/American College of Rheumatology collaborative initiative. Annals of the Rheumatic Diseases. 2012;71(4):484–492. doi:10.1136/annrheumdis-2011-200329.
13. PMRGCAuk. Polymyalgia rheumatica management guideline [Internet]. Available from: https://pmrgca.org.uk/wp-

content/uploads/2020/12/5.-Management-PMR.pdf [link to the 2010 Guideline, but soon this will be the 2026 Guideline].

14. Owen C, Lanyon P, et al. Imaging findings in polymyalgia rheumatica. Rheumatology. 2025;64(Suppl_1):i59–i63. doi:10.1093/rheumatology/keae473.
15. Fruth M, et al. MRI of the shoulder girdle in polymyalgia rheumatica: inflammatory findings and their diagnostic value. RMD Open. 2024;10:e004169. doi:10.1136/rmdopen-2024-004169.
16. Owen C, et al. Characterising polymyalgia rheumatica on whole-body 18F-FDG PET/CT: an atlas. Rheumatology Advances in Practice. 2024;8(1):rkae003. doi:10.1093/rap/rkae003.
17. Mackie SL, et al. 'An impediment to living life': why and how we should measure stiffness in polymyalgia rheumatica. PLOS One. 2015;10(5):e0126758. doi:10.1371/journal.pone.0126758.
18. Quick V, Kirwan JR. Our approach to the diagnosis and treatment of polymyalgia rheumatica and giant cell arteritis. Journal of the Royal College of Physicians of Edinburgh. 2012;42(4):341–349. doi:10.4997/JRCPE.2012.416.
19. Cowley S, et al. Real-world outcomes of a dedicated fast-track polymyalgia rheumatica clinic. Rheumatology. 2025;64(10):3006–3011.
20. Wendling D, et al. Recommendations of the French Society of Rheumatology for the management in current practice of patients with polymyalgia rheumatica. Joint Bone Spine. 2024;91(4):105730. doi:10.1016/j.jbspin.2024.105730.
21. Kay L, Lanyon P. Rheumatology: Getting It Right First Time (GIRFT) Programme National Specialty Report [Internet]. London, NHS England; 2021 [cited 2026 May 5]. Available from: https://gettingitrightfirsttime.co.uk/medical-specialties/rheumatology/
22. Tengesdal S, et al. Norwegian Society of Rheumatology recommendations on diagnosis and treatment of patients with polymyalgia rheumatica: a narrative review. BMC Rheumatology. 2024;8(1):58. doi:10.1186/s41927-024-00422-6.
23. Liew D, Owen C. Polymyalgia rheumatica: killing them softly. The Lancet Rheumatology. 2025;7:e522–e523.
24. Patil P, et al. Management of sight loss and other disease- and treatment-related complications. In: Polymyalgia rheumatica and giant cell arteritis. Oxford: Oxford University Press; 2016. p.103–118.
25. Smetana GW, Schmerling RH. Does this patient have temporal arteritis? JAMA. 2002;287(1):92–101. doi:10.1001/jama.287.1.92.

26. van der Geest K, et al. Diagnostic accuracy of symptoms, physical signs, and laboratory tests for giant cell arteritis: a systematic review and meta-analysis. JAMA Internal Medicine. 2020;180(10):1295–1304.
27. Laskou F, et al. A probability score to aid the diagnosis of suspected giant cell arteritis. Clinical and Experimental Rheumatology. 2019;37(Suppl 117):104–108.
28. Patil P, et al. Fast-track pathway reduces sight loss in giant cell arteritis. Clinical and Experimental Rheumatology. 2015;33(Suppl 89):S103–S108.
29. Diamantopoulos AP, Haugeberg G, Lindland A, Myklebust G. The fast-track ultrasound clinic for early diagnosis of giant cell arteritis significantly reduces permanent visual impairment: towards a more effective strategy to improve clinical outcome in giant cell arteritis? Rheumatology. 2016;55(1):66–70. doi:10.1093/rheumatology/kev289.
30. De Boysson H, et al. Tolerance of glucocorticoids in giant cell arteritis: a study of patient-reported adverse events. Rheumatology. 2022;61(9):3567–3575. doi:10.1093/rheumatology/keacXXX.
31. Wu J, et al. Glucocorticoid dose-dependent risk of type 2 diabetes in six immune-mediated inflammatory diseases: a population-based cohort analysis. BMJ Open Diabetes Research and Care. 2020;8(1):e001220. doi:10.1136/bmjdrc-2020-001220.
32. Pujades-Rodriguez M, et al. Dose-dependent oral glucocorticoid cardiovascular risks in people with immune-mediated inflammatory disease: a population-based cohort study. PLOS Medicine. 2020;17(12):e1003432. doi:10.1371/journal.pmed.1003432.
33. Mebrahtu TF, et al. Oral glucocorticoids and incidence of hypertension in people with chronic inflammatory diseases: a population-based cohort study. CMAJ. 2020;192:E295–E301. doi:10.1503/cmaj.191012.
34. Ducker G, et al. Adrenal insufficiency in giant cell arteritis. Rheumatology Advances in Practice. 2025;9(2):rkaf050. doi:10.1093/rap/rkaf050.
35. Hansen, SB, et al. Changes in adrenal function and insufficiency symptoms after cessation of prednisolone. JAMA Netw Open. 2025 Mar 3;8(3):e251029.
36. Beuschlein F, et al. Joint clinical guideline: diagnosis and therapy of glucocorticoid-induced adrenal insufficiency [Internet]. European Society of Endocrinology; 2024 [cited 2025 Nov 3]. Available from: https://www.ese-hormones.org/publications/directory/european-society-of-endocrinology-and-endocrine-society-joint-guideline-

diagnosis-and-therapy-of-glucocorticoid-induced-adrenal-insufficiency/

37. Mackie S, et al. British Society for Rheumatology guideline on diagnosis and treatment of giant cell arteritis: executive summary. Rheumatology. 2020;59(3):487–494. doi:10.1093/rheumatology/kez672.
38. Baker E. Is there a safe and effective way to wean patients off long-term glucocorticoids? British Journal of Clinical Pharmacology. 2021;87(1):12–22. doi:10.1111/bcp.14489.
39. Commane J, et al. A targeted literature review of the clinical and humanistic burden of polymyalgia rheumatica and the associated unmet medical needs. Annals of the Rheumatic Diseases. 2025;84(Suppl 1):2331–2332. doi:10.1016/j.ard.2025.06.2020.
40. Sattui SE, Corral M, O'Donnell DC. Illness burden and unmet patient needs in giant cell arteritis: current state and future prospects. *Open Access Rheumatol.* 2025;17:117-134. doi:10.2147/OARRR.S517664
41. Fritz S, et al. Addressing evidence gaps in polymyalgia rheumatica: findings from a literature review. Annals of the Rheumatic Diseases. 2025;84(Suppl 1)
42. Mahr AD, et al. Adjunctive methotrexate for treatment of giant cell arteritis: an individual patient data meta-analysis. Arthritis & Rheumatism. 2007;56(8):2789–2797. doi:10.1002/art.22806.
43. Koster MJ, et al. Efficacy of methotrexate in real-world management of giant cell arteritis: a case–control study. The Journal of Rheumatology. 2019;46(5):501–508. doi:10.3899/jrheum.180042.
44. Quartuccio L, et al. Faster steroid-free remission with tocilizumab compared to methotrexate in giant cell arteritis: a real-life experience in two reference centres. Rheumatology Advances in Practice. 2024;8(1):rkae0XX.
45. Kramarič J, et al. Performance of leflunomide as a steroid-sparing agent in giant cell arteritis: a single-center, open-label study. Frontiers in Medicine. 2022;9:1069013. doi:10.3389/fmed.2022.1069013.
46. Bolhuis TE, et al. PMR-MODE trial: Randomized double-blind placebo-controlled trial of methotrexate 25 mg weekly in newly diagnosed polymyalgia rheumatica. Annals of the Rheumatic Diseases. 2025;84(Suppl 1):56–57.
47. Quick V, et al. Life after tocilizumab given for giant cell arteritis: a patient survey and argument for re-treatment. Rheumatol Adv Pract. 2024;8(2):rkae054. doi:10.1093/rap/rkae054.
48. Quick V, et al. TOC STOP Study: Relapse after cessation of weekly tocilizumab for giant cell arteritis: a multicentre service evaluation

in England. Rheumatology (Oxford). 2024;63(12):3407-3414. doi:10.1093/rheumatology/kead604.

49. National Institute for Health and Care Excellence (NICE). *Tocilizumab for treating giant cell arteritis* [Internet]. London: NICE; 2018. Available from: NICE TA518 guidance.
50. Dejaco C, et al. Treat-to-target recommendations in giant cell arteritis and polymyalgia rheumatica. Annals of the Rheumatic Diseases. 2024;83(1):48–57. doi:10.1136/ard-2023-224999.
51. Muller S, et al. Characterising those with incident polymyalgia rheumatica in primary care: results from the PMR cohort study. Arthritis Research & Therapy. 2016;18(1):200. doi:10.1186/s13075-016-1097-8.
52. Tshimologo M, et al. Patients' views on the causes of their polymyalgia rheumatica: a content analysis of data from the PMR cohort study. BMC Rheumatology. 2017;1:15. doi:10.1186/s41927-017-0015-0.
53. Williams A. Women's pain is routinely underestimated, and gender stereotypes are to blame – new research [Internet]. The Conversation; 2021. Available from: https://theconversation.com/womens-pain-is-routinely-underestimated-and-gender-stereotypes-are-to-blame-new-research-158599.
54. The Sleep Charity. Sleep advice and support [Internet]. Available from: https://thesleepcharity.org.uk/.
55. Espie CA. Overcoming insomnia. London: Robinson; 2021.
56. Sleep Foundation. Sleep health information [Internet]. Available from: https://www.sleepfoundation.org/.
57. British Heart Foundation. DASH diet: foods that lower blood pressure [Internet]. Available from: https://www.bhf.org.uk/informationsupport/heart-matters-magazine/nutrition/foods-that-lower-blood-pressure/dash-diet.
58. Versus Arthritis. Arthritis information and support [Internet]. Available from: https://www.versusarthritis.org/.
59. Lerner A, et al. The effects of magnesium supplementation in autoimmune rheumatic diseases. Academia Medicine. 2024;1. doi:10.20935/AcadMed7413.
60. Heart Research Institute. Nine vegetables that are healthier for you when cooked [Internet]. Available from: https://www.hriuk.org/health/nutrition/nine-vegetables-that-are-healthier-for-you-when-cooked.
61. Esteves GP, et al. Nutritional recommendations for patients undergoing prolonged glucocorticoid therapy. Rheumatology Advances in Practice. 2022;6(2):rkac029. doi:10.1093/rap/rkac029.

62. Precision Nutrition. Elimination diet [Internet]. If you want to pursue it, detailed information on how to do the elimination diet is available from: http://www.precisionnutrition.com/elimination-diet.
63. Matei DE. Intestinal barrier dysfunction plays an integral role in arthritis pathology and can be targeted to ameliorate disease. Med. 2021;2(7):864–883.e9. doi:10.1016/j.medj.2021.04.013.
64. Carlson K, et al. Incidence of aortic aneurysm, dissection, or rupture among patients with polymyalgia rheumatica and giant cell arteritis. Semin Arthritis Rheum. 2025;72:152714. doi:10.1016/j.semarthrit.2025.152714.
65. Therkildsen P, et al. Increased risk of thoracic aortic complications among patients with giant cell arteritis: a nationwide, population-based cohort study. Rheumatology (Oxford). 2022;61(7):2931-2941. doi:10.1093/rheumatology/keab871.
66. O'Brien AV, et al. Physiotherapy for the management of polymyalgia rheumatica: results from a UK cross-sectional survey. Musculoskeletal Care. 2025:e70155. doi:10.1002/msc.70155.
67. O'Brien AV, et al. Maintaining movement, activity and exercise with PMR: a self-help guide [Internet]. Available from: Exercise-in-PMR-booklet.pdf.
68. World Health Organization. Physical activity [Internet]. Available from: https://www.who.int/news-room/fact-sheets/detail/physical-activity.
69. Age UK. Exercise and physical activity [Internet]. Available from: https://www.ageuk.org.uk/information-advice/health-wellbeing/exercise/.
70. Versus Arthritis. Exercising with arthritis [Internet]. Available from: https://www.arthritis-uk.org/information-and-support/living-with-arthritis/health-and-wellbeing/exercising-with-arthritis/ [cited 2025 Aug 28].
71. Lieber SB, et al. Frailty and rheumatic diseases: evidence to date and lessons learned. The Lancet Rheumatology. 2024;6(12):e881–e891. doi:10.1016/S2665-9913(24)00191-7.
72. Caspersen CJ, et al. Physical activity, exercise, and physical fitness: definitions and distinctions for health-related research. Public Health Reports. 1985;100(2):126–131. PMID:3920711.
73. Yerrakalva D, et al. Associations between change in physical activity and sedentary time and health-related quality of life in older English adults: the EPIC-Norfolk cohort study. Health and Quality of Life Outcomes. 2023;21:137. doi:10.1186/s12955-023-02137-7.
74. Leung JL, De Ross B, Gianoudis J, Deeble N, Yang V, Azzopardi R, et al. More than pain and stiffness: persistent fatigue and sleep disturbance characterise polymyalgia rheumatica. *J Rheumatol.* 2025;52(7):704-712. doi:10.3899/jrheum.2024-0980.

75. Dures E, et al. 2023 EULAR recommendations for the management of fatigue in people with inflammatory rheumatic and musculoskeletal diseases. Annals of the Rheumatic Diseases. 2024;83:1260–1267. doi:10.1136/ard-2023-224514.
76. Chatzigeorgiou C, Mackie SL. Comorbidity in polymyalgia rheumatica. Reumatismo. 2018;70(1):35–43. doi:10.4081/reumatismo.2018.1039.
77. National Institute for Health and Care Excellence. Corticosteroids: general use [Internet]. London: NICE; 2025 [cited 2025 Jun 3]. Available from: https://bnf.nice.org.uk/treatment-summaries/corticosteroids-general-use/
78. Hider S, et al. People with polymyalgia rheumatica need a falls assessment and regular treatment reviews. NIHR Evidence [Internet]. 2022 [cited 2025 Aug 21]. Available from: https://doi.org/10.3310/nihrevidence_51304.
79. NHS. Physical activity guidelines for older adults [Internet]. 2025 [cited 2025 Aug 28]. Available from: https://www.nhs.uk/live-well/exercise/physical-activity-guidelines-older-adults/
80. Mackie S, et al. National Institute for Health and Care Research. The polymyalgia paradox: Addressing north-south inequities in polymyalgia rheumatica using grassroots community connectors in a deprived urban area [version 1; not peer reviewed]. NIHR Open Res. 2025;5:122. doi:10.3310/nihropenres.1115283.1.
81. Muller S, et al. Support available for and perceived priorities of people with polymyalgia rheumatica and giant cell arteritis: results of the PMRGCAuk members' survey 2017. Clinical Rheumatology. 2018;37(12):3411–3418. doi:10.1007/s10067-018-4220-1.

Acknowledgements

A book is never the work of a single person, and in this case, Vanessa and I are grateful for the support of many people. To begin with, I want to thank the team at PMRGCAuk for their enthusiasm for the project and practical help. Sophie Boyce and Sir Humphrey Hodgson were key at the start when I tentatively approached the charity about a new edition. Thanks to them I was able to access the information and resources I needed to get started. Fran Benson, Fiona Johnson and Janette Manelle have continued to be stalwart supporters and spread the word that the third edition was on its way.

Dr Sarah Mackie gave me encouragement from the medical side and pointed me towards what she felt was most important, with her extraordinary sensitivity to the burden of PMR and GCA on people's lives. Thanks also go to the people who generously shared their stories; Penny Denby and members of Kent support group; Gail Booth and the Cheshire group; Val, Jeff, Carole, Shirley, Eileen, Alec, Lynda, Stella, Lil, Julianne, Pam, Fressia, A, OxfordBoy2; everyone on HealthUnlocked; Duane Mellor; Anne O'Brien for the chapter, and Matthew Baxter for the illustrations; and every rheumatologist who ever taught me just by having a great conversation.

Huge thanks to Eileen, Fiona, Sarah, and Fran for their critical read of the manuscript, and to Anne Fox for her eagle-eyed proofreading. Andy O'Dwyer (www.andyodwyer.com) has done a brilliant job of the cover design.

But most of all, the biggest thanks go to my amazing co-author, Vanessa, who took a huge leap of faith, and has bravely and selflessly shared her knowledge and experience as a rheumatologist. She has enriched every part of this book. Vanessa, you have been a joy to work with, and I will treasure the experience of working with you for the rest of my life. Without you, this could never have happened.

About the authors

Dr Kate Gilbert PhD was a successful head of department in a UK business school when she became ill with polymyalgia rheumatica. She went on to help set up the UK charity PMRGCAuk and served on the board of trustees for six years. Her experience of teaching research methods to Masters students honed her skill for explaining complex concepts to non-medical people, and she distilled what she had learned from working alongside rheumatologists and researchers into this 'survival guide'. She lives in the English Midlands with her husband and cats, and spends as much time as possible on her allotment. Contact Kate on polywotsit@gmail.com.

Dr Vanessa Quick MBBS MRCP FHEA is a Consultant Rheumatologist and GCA Lead at Bedfordshire Hospitals NHS Foundation Trust in the South of England. Alongside her clinical work, she is involved in medical education, research, and service development of fast-track pathways for patients with GCA and PMR. Through her work as a Trustee of PMRGCAuk, she has developed a particular interest in making medical information more understandable and accessible to those living with these conditions. She lives with her husband and two teenage children and especially enjoys family holidays by, or preferably on, the sea.

www.ingramcontent.com/pod-product-compliance
Ingram Content Group UK Ltd.
Pitfield, Milton Keynes, MK11 3LW, UK
UKHW020123290926
15471UKWH00003B/245

9 781066 664603